Textbook of
RADIOLOGY
Physics

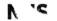

Textbook of
RADIOLOGY
Physics

Editors

Hariqbal Singh MD DMRD
Professor and Head
Department of Radiology
Shrimati Kashibai Navale Medical College and General Hospital
Pune, Maharashtra, India

Amol Sasane MD
Lecturer
Department of Radiology
Shrimati Kashibai Navale Medical College and General Hospital
Pune, Maharashtra, India

Roshan Lodha DMRD
Consultant
Department of Radiology
Shrimati Kashibai Navale Medical College and General Hospital
Pune, Maharashtra, India

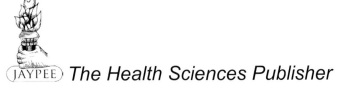

JAYPEE *The Health Sciences Publisher*

New Delhi | London | Philadelphia | Panama

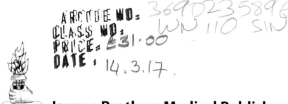

Jaypee Brothers Medical Publishers (P) Ltd.

Headquarters

Jaypee Brothers Medical Publishers (P) Ltd.
4838/24, Ansari Road, Daryaganj
New Delhi 110 002, India
Phone: +91-11-43574357
Fax: +91-11-43574314
E-mail: jaypee@jaypeebrothers.com

Overseas Offices

J.P. Medical Ltd.
83, Victoria Street, London
SW1H 0HW (UK)
Phone: +44 20 3170 8910
Fax: +44(0) 20 3008 6180
E-mail: info@jpmedpub.com

Jaypee Highlights Medical Publishers Inc.
City of Knowledge, Building 235, 2nd Floor
Clayton, Panama City, Panama
Phone: +1 507-301-0496
Fax: +1 507-301-0499
E-mail: cservice@jphmedical.com

Jaypee Medical Inc.
325, Chestnut Street
Suite 412, Philadelphia, PA 19106, USA
Phone: +1 267-519-9789
E-mail: support@jpmedus.com

Jaypee Brothers Medical Publishers (P) Ltd.
17/1-B, Babar Road, Block-B, Shaymali
Mohammadpur, Dhaka-1207
Bangladesh
Mobile: +08801912003485
E-mail: jaypeedhaka@gmail.com

Jaypee Brothers Medical Publishers (P) Ltd.
Bhotahity, Kathmandu, Nepal
Phone: +977-9741283608
E-mail: kathmandu@jaypeebrothers.com

Website: www.jaypeebrothers.com
Website: www.jaypeedigital.com

Inquiries for bulk sales may be solicited at: jaypee@jaypeebrothers.com

Textbook of Radiology: Physics

First Edition: **2016**

ISBN: 978-93-85891-30-4

Printed at Sanat Printers

Dedicated to

Students and teachers involved in
professional programs and work in diagnostic radiology

Saying

In physics, questioning should not halt,
curiosity must not extinct,
comprehend the mysteries of eternity, life, and amazing composition of reality,
grasp a little of this mystery each day.

Hariqbal Singh

Contributors

Aditi Dongre MD (Radiology)
Associate Professor
Department of Radiology
Shrimati Kashibai Navale Medical College and
General Hospital
Pune, Maharashtra, India

Amol Sasane MD
Lecturer
Department of Radiology
Shrimati Kashibai Navale Medical College and
General Hospital
Pune, Maharashtra, India

Anand Kamat MD (Radiology)
Professor
Department of Radiology
Shrimati Kashibai Navale Medical College and
General Hospital
Pune, Maharashtra, India

Chandan Mishra MBBS
Clinical Research Calibrator
Siemens
Mumbai, Maharashtra, India

Hariqbal Singh MD DMRD
Professor and Head
Department of Radiology
Shrimati Kashibai Navale Medical College and
General Hospital
Pune, Maharashtra, India

Manisha Hadgaonkar DNB
Assistant Professor
Department of Radiology
Shrimati Kashibai Navale Medical College and
General Hospital
Pune, Maharashtra, India

Parvez Seikh DMRE
Consultant
Department of Radiology
Shrimati Kashibai Navale Medical College and
General Hospital
Pune, Maharashtra, India

Prashant Naik MD (Radiology)
Associate Professor
Department of Radiology
Shrimati Kashibai Navale Medical College and
General Hospital
Pune, Maharashtra, India

Rajlaxmi Sharma DMRE
Consultant
Department of Radiology
Shrimati Kashibai Navale Medical College and
General Hospital
Pune, Maharashtra, India

Raunaklaxmi Laul DNB (Radiology)
Consultant
Department of Radiology
Shrimati Kashibai Navale Medical College and
General Hospital
Pune, Maharashtra, India

Roshan Lodha DMRD
Consultant
Department of Radiology
Shrimati Kashibai Navale Medical College and
General Hospital
Pune, Maharashtra, India

Santosh Konde MD (Radiology)
Associate Professor
Department of Radiology
Shrimati Kashibai Navale Medical College and
General Hospital
Pune, Maharashtra, India

Shailendra Savale MBBS
Consultant
Department of Radiology
Shrimati Kashibai Navale Medical College and
General Hospital
Pune, Maharashtra, India

Shrikant Nagare DNB (Radiology)
Consultant
Department of Radiology
Shrimati Kashibai Navale Medical College and
General Hospital
Pune, Maharashtra, India

Sikandar Shaikh DMRD DNB EDiR (European Board of Radiology)
Consultant
Department of Radiology and PET-CT
Yashoda Hospitals
Hyderabad, Telangana, India

Subodh Laul DNB
Consultant
Department of Radiology
Shrimati Kashibai Navale Medical College and
General Hospital
Pune, Maharashtra, India

Sujit Nilagaonkar DRM DNB
Consultant (Nuclear Medicine)
Shrimati Kashibai Navale Medical College and
General Hospital
Pune, Maharashtra, India

Varsha Rangankar MD (Radiology)
Associate Professor
Department of Radiology
Shrimati Kashibai Navale Medical College and
General Hospital
Pune, Maharashtra, India

Yasmeen Khan DMRE
Consultant
Department of Radiology
Shrimati Kashibai Navale Medical College and
General Hospital
Pune, Maharashtra, India

Preface

Physics is the scientific study of matter and energy and how they interact with each other. Energy can take the form of motion, light, electricity, radiation, or gravity, or just about anything. Physics deals with matter on scales ranging from sub-atomic particles to stars and galaxies.

Clinical or medical physicists engage with areas of testing, optimization, quality assurance of diagnostic equipment including X-rays, fluoroscopy, mammography, angiography, computed tomography, ultrasound, magnetic resonance imaging (MRI), radiation exposure monitoring, dosimetry, nuclear medicine, single-photon emission computed tomography (SPECT), and positron emission tomography (PET).

This book is to-the-point and keeping the length limited, developed especially for students of radiology preparing for examination and who are always short of time. It is not intended to be a comprehensive reference. It teaches the essential physics of diagnostic radiology and its application in modern medicine. It is structured such that the student is pioneered to radiology physics and is prepared to do well in examination without taking surplus time. Adequate figures and tables have been endowed with to give a better understanding of the subject. The book covers most questions asked in and during theory and practical examination.

The book is meant for radiology residents, radiologists and technical staff of any imaging institute. It is meant for medical colleges, institutional and departmental libraries.

Hariqbal Singh
Amol Sasane
Roshan Lodha

Acknowledgments

We express thanks designed for Professor MN Navale, Founder President, Sinhgad Technical Educational Society and Dr Arvind V Bhore, Dean, Shrimati Kashibai Navale Medical College and General Hospital, for their kind assent in this venture.

We are profusely gratified to the radiology residents Swati Shah, Vikram Shende, Jarvis Pereira, Priya Bhole, Prasad Patil, Punit Agrawal, Swapnil Raut, Amar Sangapwad, and Prajakta Jagtap, for their genuine help in correction of the manuscript.

Our special thanks to our Artist-cum-Photographer Manoj Nalawade and Sanjay Raut for developing on most images.

Our gratitude to Shankar Gopale, Anna Bansode, Sachin Babar, and Snehal Bhairamadgikar, for their untiring clerical help.

We appreciate Kavita Mangotra, Manager, Clinical Applications, Siemens Ltd, for providing information on wireless transducers.

This book is a compilation developed by unified, consistent and cohesive endeavor of the panel of radiologists at Shrimati Kashibai Navale Medical College and General Hospital, Pune, Maharashtra, India.

We are thankful and grateful to God Almighty and mankind who have allowed us to have this wonderful experience.

Contents

PLATE 1

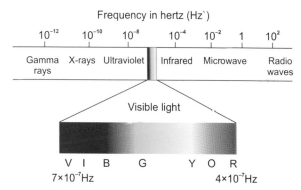

Fig. 1.1 Electromagnetic spectrum showing frequency of various electromagnetic radiations

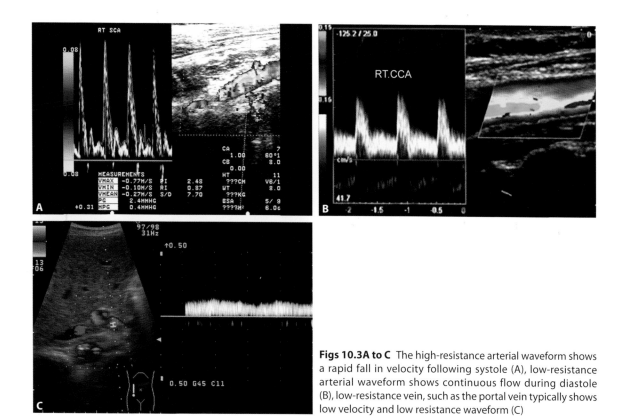

Figs 10.3A to C The high-resistance arterial waveform shows a rapid fall in velocity following systole (A), low-resistance arterial waveform shows continuous flow during diastole (B), low-resistance vein, such as the portal vein typically shows low velocity and low resistance waveform (C)

Fig. 10.4B Typical spectral waveform pattern with parameter display

PLATE 2

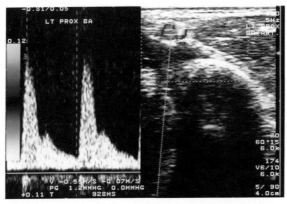

Fig. 10.6 Spectral broadening occurs due to mixture of large number of different velocities in a sample volume with filling—in of the "window" under the spectral curve

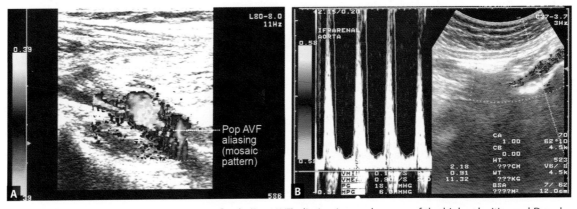

Figs 10.7A and B (A) Popliteal arteriovenous fistula (Pop AVF)-aliasing is seen because of the high velocities and Doppler shift frequencies are above the Nyquist limit. Aliasing is seen as a color change from red through yellow, to blue giving 'mosaic pattern' on color flow imaging; (B) Aortic stenosis- In Doppler waveform the peak velocity is cut off and the high frequencies "wrap around" and are displayed on the opposite side of the baseline

PLATE 3

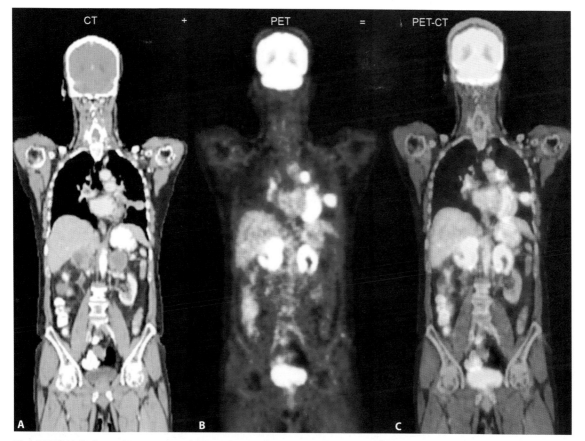

Figs 18.1A to C Coronal reconstructed CT image: (A) of thorax and abdomen showing mass in lung and mass lesion in both adrenals. Post FDG injection PET; (B) and fused PET-CT; (C) image shows increased tracer uptake in lung mass and bilateral adrenals, suggestive of carcinoma lung with adrenal metastases

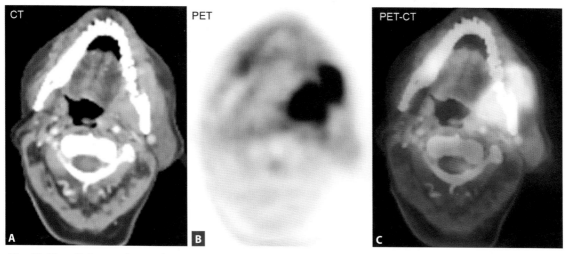

Figs 18.2A to C Operated case of tongue carcinoma, axial CT shows a lesion (A) There is intense tracer uptake suggestive of recurrence of tumor (B, C)

PLATE 4

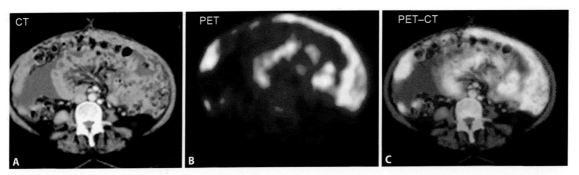

Figs 18.3A to C Axial CT image in the case of Ca ovary with multiple peritoneal deposits. Mild ascites also noted; (A) Post FDG injection PET; (B) and PET-CT; (C) image shows increased tracer uptake suggestive of peritoneal metastases

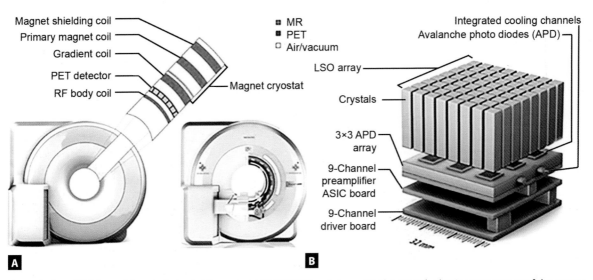

Figs 19.1A and B View of the whole-body Biograph mMR, MR-PET prototype: (A) Showing the basic components of the system where the PET detector ring is placed between the RF coil and the RF body coil; (B) Configuration of the detector block consisting of 8×8 LSO crystals read-out by a matrix of 3×3 APDs. LSO is Lutetium Oxyorthosilicate and ASIC is detector stack

PLATE 5

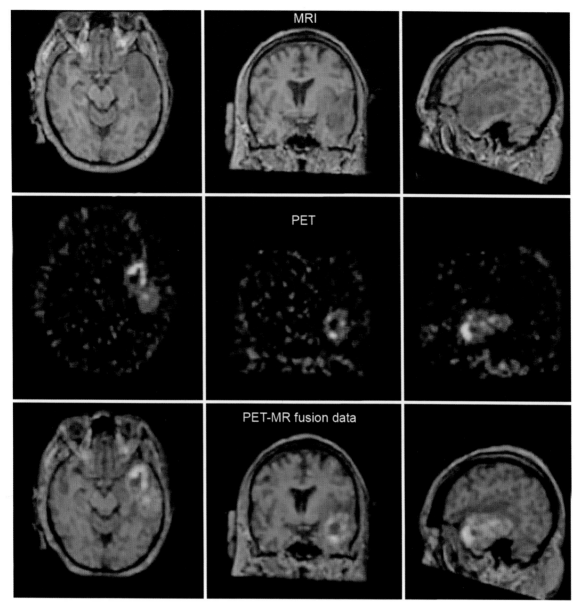

Fig. 19.2 MR, PET and fusion images demonstrates the glioma proliferation (*Courtesy:* Siemens AG, Germany)

PLATE 6

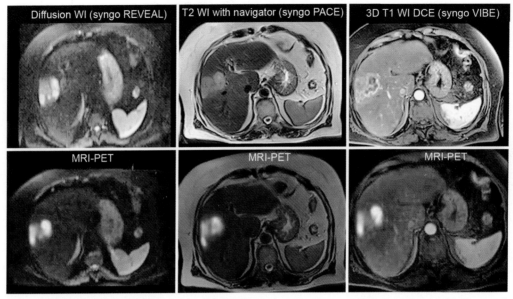

Fig. 19.3 Simultaneous acquisition PET with multiple MRI information showing better characterization of hepatic lesion

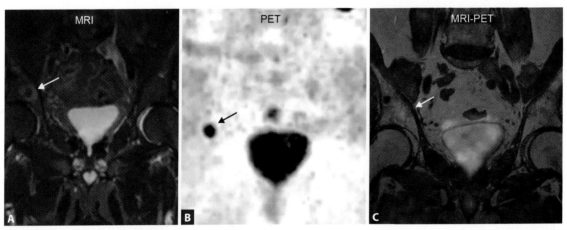

Figs 19.4A to C Simultaneous MR and PET support detection and monitoring of prostate cancer where whole-body MR offers high contrast to identify small and diffuse metastasis and PET enables superb lesion detection and differentiation (A) whole body MR; (B) Choline PET; (C) simultaneous MR and PET

PLATE 7

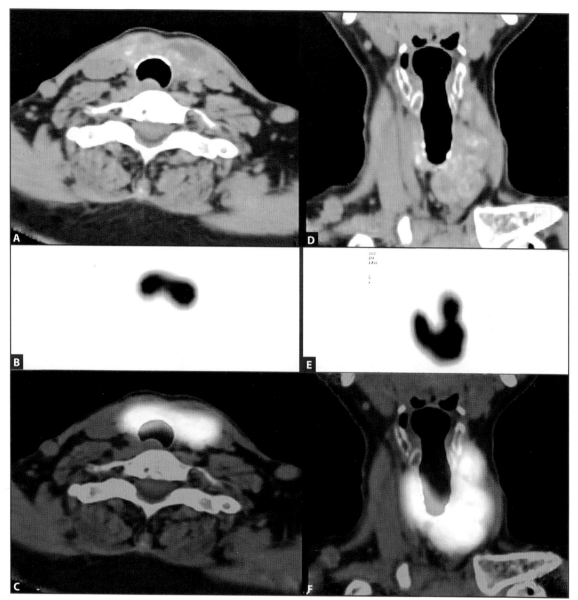

Figs 20.1A to F Axial and coronal CT images of neck (A and D) showing multiple nodules in both lobes of thyroid, more on the left. On administration of 131I, it shows increased uptake in thyroid gland seen on fusion images of SPECT (B, C, E and F)

PLATE 8

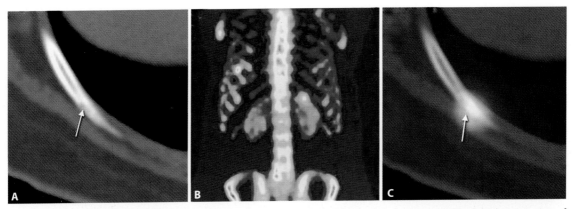

Figs 20.2A to C Axial CT image of thorax on bone window shows a suspicious lytic lesion in rib (A). On administration of Technetium-99m methylene diphosphonate (MDP) it showed increased uptake in rib, seen on fusion images suggestive of metastatic lesion (B and C)

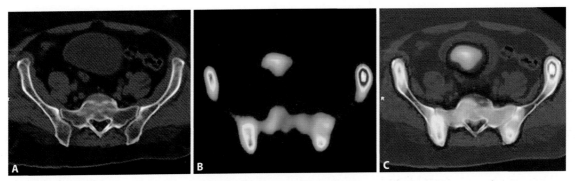

Figs 20.3A to C Axial CT section at level of iliac bones does not show any obvious abnormality in a case of prostate cancer (A). On administration of 111In capromab pendetide it showed increased uptake in prostate gland and left anterior superior iliac spine, seen on fusion images, s/o metastatic lesion (B and C)

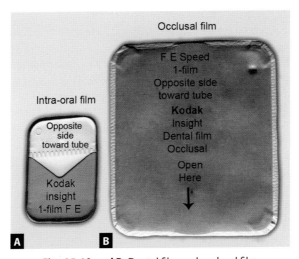

Figs 25.4A and B Dental film and occlusal film

1
Electromagnetic Radiations

Shrikant Nagare

In 1820, Hans Oersted (Denmark) and Andre Marie Ampere (France) found that conductor carrying electric current produces magnetism. In 1831, Michel Faraday of England and Joseph Henry of USA discovered that magnetism produces electric current by electromagnetic induction. In 1864 Clerk Maxwell of England showed that electric and magnetic fields together produce radiant energy in the form of electromagnetic waves. In 1880, Heinrich Hertz of Germany verified Maxwell's predictions and discovered radio waves.

In 1895, Wilhelm Conrad Roentgen of Germany discovered X-rays. They are a form of electromagnetic radiation (EMR) with a wavelength in the range of 10 to 0.01 nanometers. Their wavelength is longer than Gamma rays but shorter than Ultraviolet rays. Roentgen, while investigating cathode rays from a Crookes tube wrapped in black cardboard in a darkened room to block visible light, noticed a faint green glow from the fluorescent screen painted with barium platinocyanide, about a meter away. The invisible rays were passing through the cardboard. Roentgen discovered its medical use when he saw on 22 December 1895 the picture of his wife Anna Bertha's hand on a photographic plate formed due to X-rays. That was the first ever radiograph of a human body part.

Radioactivity is characterized by a transformation of an unstable nucleus into a more stable entity that may be unstable and will decay further through a chain of decays until a stable nuclear configuration is reached. Radiation is direct transmission of heat or electromagnetic energy through space or another medium.

Electromagnetic radiation is a combination of oscillating electric and magnetic fields propagating perpendicular to each other through space and carrying energy stored in the propagating wave, from one place to another. It is like a sinusoidal variation of electric and magnetic fields in space. Its velocity is about 300,000 km/sec in space. Light is a form of EMR.

PROPERTIES OF ELECTROMAGNETIC RADIATION

Electromagnetic radiation of all wave lengths or frequencies travels in straight lines with the same velocity in free space, transfer energy from place to place in form of quanta. While passing through matter the intensity of the radiation is reduced due to absorption and scattering.

CLASSIFICATION OF RADIATION

- Ionizing radiation is classified into directly ionizing (charged particles like electrons and protons) and indirectly ionizing radiation (photons, e.g. X-rays, gamma rays and neutrons). Directly ionizing radiations deposit energy in the medium through the interaction between the directly ionized charged particle and orbital electrons of the atoms in the medium. Indirectly ionizing radiations deposit energy in the medium by a two step process:
    1. Release of a charged particle in the medium (e.g. photons release electrons/positrons, neutrons release protons).
    2. Released charged particles deposit energy in the medium by interacting with the orbital electrons of the atoms.
- Nonionizing radiations refer to electromagnetic radiation that does not carry enough energy per quantum to ionize atoms or molecules. Near ultraviolet, visible light, infrared, microwave and radio waves are all examples of nonionizing radiation.

IONIZING RADIATION

When a stable atom either loses or gains an electron and becomes unstable it is called an ion. A photon of 15 electron volt (eV) or more of energy is capable of ionizing the atoms and molecules. Gamma rays, X-rays and a few ultraviolet rays are ionizing radiations. X-rays are produced when electrons, traveling at high speed, collide with a target material, such as tungsten. The kinetic energy of the electrons is converted into electromagnetic radiation. Part of this radiation is X-rays. X-rays and other types of electromagnetic radiation are emitted as small packets of electromagnetic energy called photons. A photon is characterized by the electromagnetic wavelength. X-rays are produced in an X-ray tube which consists of a vacuum glass envelope in which a filament and a target are placed. The vacuum is needed so that electrons emitted from the filament can move freely to the target material. The filament is the cathode. The target material is the anode. If the filament is heated, electrons are emitted. The higher the temperature of the filament, the more electrons are emitted. An X-ray beam consists of different wavelengths and beam is called a polychromatic beam.

Interaction of high speed electrons with target decides the type of radiation produced. Interaction with nucleus causes no ionization and produces bremsstrahlung (general) radiation. Interaction with shell electrons causes ionization of atoms in target and produces characteristic radiation.

Electromagnetic energy travels in the form of waves. The waves have high points (crests) and the low points (troughs). The maximum height of the wave from its equilibrium position is called as the amplitude of the wave. The distance between two consecutive crests or troughs, or distance covered by one full crest and one full trough is known as wavelength. The symbol for wavelength is the Greek letter lambda (λ). Another important parameter of wave discussion is frequency of the wave (f). Frequency of the wave represents the number of waves that pass a given point per second. The unit of frequency is Hertz (Hz). Speed at which a wave travels through a medium is known as wave speed or wave velocity (v). Wave speed, frequency and wavelength together form an important equation called general wave equation,

Wave speed (v) = wavelength (λ) × frequency (f).

The electromagnetic spectrum (Fig. 1.1) is the range of all possible frequencies of electromagnetic radiation. They are broadly classified as

- *Gamma radiation:* Gamma rays originate from the nucleus of an unstable (i.e. radioactive) atom. Radioactive materials that emit these types of penetrating radiations find use in nuclear medicine department.
- *X-rays:* X-rays occupy same portion of electromagnetic spectrum as gamma rays, only

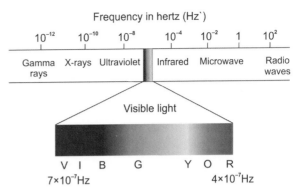

Fig. 1.1 Electromagnetic spectrum showing frequency of various electromagnetic radiations (*For color version, see Plate 1*)

difference being their origin. X-rays originate from outside the nucleus of atom and gamma rays originate from within the nucleus. At higher intensities X-rays can produce skin burns and lead to more serious biological complications. At lower intensities X-rays are used for radiography.

- *Ultraviolet radiation:* Ultraviolet radiation is the band of wavelengths just beyond the visible spectrum. It has energy more than visible light.
- *Visible light:* Visible light is that portion of electromagnetic radiation which can be appreciated by human eyes. Wavelengths corresponding to various colors of visible light are ranging from 700 nm to 400 nm. Visible light occupies very small portion of electromagnetic spectrum.
- *Infrared radiations:* These radiations comprise of wavelengths which are just longer than the longest portion of visible spectrum.
- *Microwaves:* Microwaves consist of the waves from the electromagnetic spectrum with frequencies ranging from 1 to 30 Ghz. Previously microwaves have been used in radar and satellite communications. Microwaves are used in the field of medicine for deep tissue heating and treatment of certain type of cancers in conjunction with other modes of therapy. This mode of treatment is referred to as microwave diathermy. Microwaves have also been used in linear accelerators in radiation therapy departments.
- *Radio waves:* These are comprised of wide range of frequencies from (20 kHz to 1 GHz) and these are used in aircraft and marine navigation, radio transmissions and television broadcasts. Frequencies in lower megahertz range correspond to those currently used in magnetic resonance imaging (MRI).

2

Production of X-ray

Yasmeen Khan

X-rays are produced by sudden stoppage of rapidly moving high energy electrons. The source of electrons is the cathode, or negative electrode. Electrons are stopped or decelerated by the anode, or positive electrode. The potential charge difference between the electrodes accelerates electrons from cathode to anode (Fig. 2.1).

Cathode is a negatively charged electrode made up of a coiled thin tungsten wire. Cathode is also known as filament which is fitted in a focusing cup made of nickel. Filament serves as the source of electrons during X-ray production. Focusing cup surrounds the filament to focus the stream of electrons before they strike the anode. Most X-ray tubes use two filaments; a large and a small. Only one filament is used at any one time during X-ray production.

Anode is a positively charged electrode. The small area on anode which receives a high energy electron beam from cathode is known as target. The target stops the electrons and produces X-rays. There are two types of anodes; stationary anode (Fig. 2.2) and rotating anode (Fig. 2.3). The target is made of tungsten (90%) and rhenium (10%) alloy. Tungsten is used as the material of choice because of its high atomic number of 74 and a high melting point of 3370°C.

The X-ray tube housing is made up of a Pyrex glass containing a vacuum. A potential difference or voltage is applied between the cathode and anode. The tungsten filament (cathode) is heated by an independent current to emit electrons; a process called thermionic emission. The focusing cup directs the emitted electrons across the vacuum to hit the small spot (focal spot) on the anode target. The electrons that hit the tungsten target undergo sudden deflection because of the interactions with the tungsten nucleus. The tungsten target is usually angled (6 to 20°) to direct the resultant X-rays towards a window in the tube wall. The window is thin and made of glass. In mammography units the window is made of beryllium. There is generation of heat from the anode. To dissipate the heat generated there is oil based cooling system surrounding the anode. Rotating anode tubes have a spinning electrode (3,300 rpm to 10,000 rpm) to effectively increase the surface area.

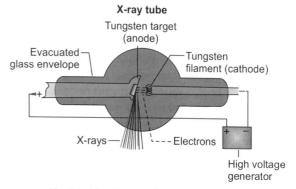

Fig. 2.1 Line diagram showing structure of stationary X-ray tube

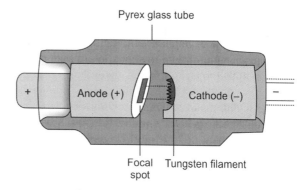

Fig. 2.2 Stationary anode X-ray tube

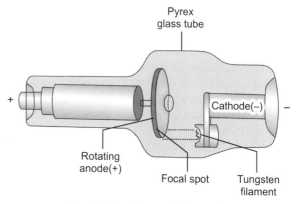

Fig. 2.3 Rotating anode X-ray tube

X-rays are produced in all directions from focal spot, but beam restriction devices (e.g. collimators) are used to allow only a primary beam to escape the source and irradiate the patient.

MECHANISM OF X-RAY PRODUCTION

There are two main mechanisms of X-ray production. One involves reaction of the high speed electrons with the nucleus of the tungsten atoms, producing X-rays that are termed general radiation, or bremsstrahlung. The second involves collision between the high speed electrons and the electrons in the shell of the target tungsten atoms, producing X-rays that are called characteristic radiation.

- *General radiation or bremsstrahlung (which in German means breaking radiation):* When high speed electron passes near the nucleus of a tungsten atom, the positive charge of the nucleus attracts the negative charged electron. The electron is deflected from its original direction. The electron lose energy and slowed down when its direction changes. The kinetic energy lost by the electron is emitted directly in the form of a photon of radiation. The radiation produced by this process is called general radiation or bremsstrahlung (Fig. 2.4).
  The energy of the emitted X-ray photon resulting from deceleration of electrons in the electric field of a nucleus depends on how close the electron passes to the nucleus, the energy of the electron, and the charge of the nucleus.
- *Characteristic radiation:* Characteristic radiation results when the electrons bombarding the target eject electrons from the inner orbits of the target atoms (A in Fig. 2.5). When an electron is ejected from an atom, the vacancy in the electron shell is filled by another electron from one of the electron shells farther out from the nucleus (B in Fig. 2.5). Following this process, the atom contains excess energy. This excess energy can be emitted in two

ways; either by pushing out one of the loosest bound electrons in the outermost shell or by emitting an X-ray photon. The electrons emitted are called Auger electrons, and the photons emitted are called characteristic radiation. A tungsten atom with an inner shell vacancy is much more likely to produce an X-ray than to expel an electron.

The higher the atomic number of the target atoms, the greater will be the efficiency of the production of X-rays. The atomic number of the target material determines the quantity (number) of bremsstrahlung produced and determines the quality (energy) of the characteristic radiation.

The energy of the electrons is determined by the peak kilo voltage (kVp) used. Therefore, the kVp determines the maximum energy (quality/penetration) of the X-rays produced. In addition, higher kVp techniques will also increase the quantity of X-rays produced.

The number of X-rays produced depends on the number of electrons that strike the target of the anode. The number of electrons depends directly on the tube current (mA) applied. The greater the mA the more electrons that are produced; consequently, more X-rays will be produced. The current (mA) applied for a time period in seconds, i.e. milliampere-seconds (mAs) determines the radiographic film blackening.

Characteristics of X-rays

- They are invisible to human eyes.
- They are electrically neutral. They have neither a positive nor a negative charge. They cannot be accelerated or made to change direction by a magnet or electrical field.
- They have no mass.
- They travel in a straight line at the speed of light in vacuum.
- They form a polyenergetic beam.

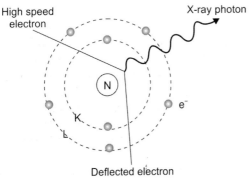

Fig. 2.4 The production of general radiation (bremsstrahlung)

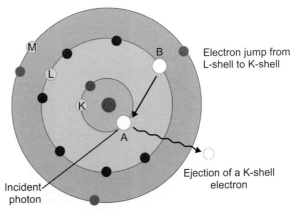

Fig. 2.5 The production of characteristic radiation

- The X-ray beam used in diagnostic radiography comprises many photons that have much different energy.
- They cause fluorescence in some substances.
- They cause chemical changes in radiographic and photographic film.
- They are absorbed or scattered by tissues in the human body.
- They produce secondary radiation.
- They cause chemical and biologic damage to living tissue.

ROTATING ANODE

With the development of powerful X-ray generators the limiting factor in the X-ray output becomes the X-ray tube itself. The ability of the X-ray tube to achieve high X-ray outputs is limited by the heat generated at the anode. To overcome this, rotating anode principle is used to produce X-ray tubes capable of withstanding the heat generated by large exposures.

The anode of a rotating anode tube consists of a large disc of tungsten, or an alloy of tungsten, which theoretically rotates at a speed of about 3600 revolutions per minute (Fig. 2.6) when an exposure is being made. The purpose of the rotating anode is to spread the heat produced during an exposure over a large area of the anode.

The power to effect rotation is provided by a magnetic field produced by stator coils that surround the neck of the X-ray tube outside the envelope. The magnetic field produced by the stator coils induces a current in the copper rotor of the induction motor, and this induced current provides the power to rotate the anode assembly. Heat generated in a solid tungsten disc is dissipated by radiating through the vacuum to the wall of the tube, and then into the surrounding oil and tube housing. In the rotating anode tube, absorption of heat by the anode assembly is undesirable because heat absorbed by the bearings of the anode assembly would cause them to expand and bind. Because of this

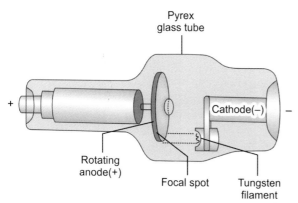

Fig. 2.6 Rotating anode X-ray tube

problem the stem, which connects the tungsten target to the remainder of the anode assembly, is made of molybdenum. Molybdenum has a high melting point (2600°C) and is a relatively poor heat conductor. Thus, the molybdenum stem provides a partial heat barrier between the tungsten disc and the bearings of the anode assembly.

The length of the molybdenum stem should be kept as short as possible to decrease the load on the bearings of the anode assembly. This problem is reduced in metal tubes by the use of bearings at each end of the anode axle.

Working of a Rotating Anode Tube

During exposure the anode rotates rapidly while being bombarded by the electron stream. During rotation, the anode constantly turns a new face to the electron beam so that the heating effect of the beam does not concentrate at one focus point as in a stationary anode, but spreads over a large area called the focal track. But the effective focus remains constant in position relative to the film because of the extremely smooth motion of the anode.

TRANSFORMER

High Tension Transformer

High tension transformer is a new type of transformer which uses the principle of high-frequency current to produce an almost constant potential voltage to the X-ray tube.

A transformer is a device that either increases or decreases the voltage in a circuit. The X-ray generator receives 115- or 230-V, 60-Hz (cycles per second) alternating current. Filament heating requires a potential difference of approximately 10 V, whereas electron acceleration requires a potential difference that can be varied between 40,000 and 150,000 V. Transformers are used to change the potential difference of the incoming electric energy to the appropriate level.

A transformer consists of two wire coils wrapped around a closed core (Fig. 2.7). The core may be a simple rectangle with the windings wound around opposite sides of the rectangle. The circuit containing the first coil (which is connected to the available electric energy source) is called the primary circuit, and the circuit containing the second coil (from which comes the modified electric energy) is called the secondary circuit.

The core of a transformer is laminated. It is made up of thin sheets of special iron alloys separated from each other by thin insulating layers. The purpose of the

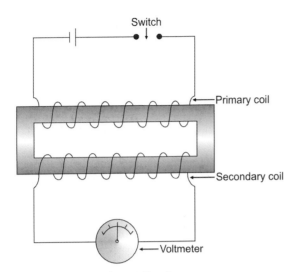

Fig. 2.7 Transformer

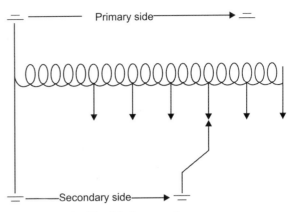

Fig. 2.8 Autotransformer

laminations is to reduce eddy currents, which waste power and appear as heat in the transformer core.

The basic principle involved is this: In a transformer, the voltage induced in the secondary coil is proportional to the rate of change of current in the primary coil.

The incoming power supply is standard 60-Hz current. The current is rectified and smoothed. This direct current is then fed to a device, often called a chopper, which converts the smoothed DC into a chopped DC with a frequency of about 6500 Hz. This 6500-Hz chopped DC supplies the primary of a step-up transformer, which steps up the voltage. The high voltage 6500-Hz output of the transformer is rectified to produce 13,000 high-voltage pulses per second, and then smoothened by filters before being applied to the X-ray tube. This provides voltage to the X-ray tube that is nearly ripple-free. It supplies a constant, nearly ripple-free voltage to the X-ray tube regardless of the input power. No special power supply or voltage regulators are required. Another advantage is the very small size of these generators.

The output is determined by the rate of change of flux, and is proportional to the frequency, the number of windings in the secondary, and the cross-sectional area of the core.

V = fnA (output voltage = frequency X number of windings X core cross-sectional area)

V = output voltage
f = frequency
n = number of windings
A = core cross-sectional area

We can maintain a constant output voltage by increasing the frequency and decreasing the number of turns or the core cross-sectional area.

AUTOTRANSFORMER

It is an electromagnetic device which operates on the principle of self induction. The auto prefix refers to the single coil acting on itself rather than any automatic mechanism. A single coil or winding serves as the primary and secondary coil (Fig. 2.8), the number of turns being adjustable. The winding has at least three taps where electrical connections are made. The ratio of voltage output to voltage input can be varied by varying the number of turns in the primary and secondary coil.

This principle is governed by the *autotransformer law.*

$$\frac{\text{Autotransformer secondary voltage}}{\text{Autotransformer primary voltage}} = \frac{\text{Number of secondary turns}}{\text{Number of primary turns}}$$

Functions of Autotransformers

- Provides voltage for the X-ray tube filament circuit
- Provides voltage for the primary of the high-voltage transformer
- Provides suitable voltage for subsidiary circuits, which we will not consider
- Provides a convenient location for the kVp meter that indicates the voltage to be applied across the X-ray tube.

Working of an Autotransformer

An autotransformer has a single winding with two end terminals, and one or more terminals at intermediate tap points. The primary voltage is applied across two of the terminals, and the secondary voltage taken from two terminals, almost always having one terminal in common with the primary voltage. The primary and secondary circuits therefore have a number of windings turns in common. Since the volts-per-turn is the same in both windings, each develops a voltage in proportion to its number of turns. In an autotransformer part of the current flows directly from the input to the output, and only part is transferred inductively, allowing a smaller, lighter, cheaper core to be used as well as requiring only a single winding.

One end of the winding is usually connected in common to both the voltage source and the electrical load. The other end of the source and load are connected to taps along the winding. Different taps on the winding correspond to different voltages, measured from the common end. In a step-down transformer the source is usually connected across the entire winding while the load is connected by a tap across only a portion of the winding. In a step-up transformer, conversely, the load is attached across the full winding while the source is connected to a tap across a portion of the winding.

As in a two-winding transformer, the ratio of secondary to primary voltages is equal to the ratio of the number of turns of the winding they connect to. For example, connecting the load between the middle and bottom of the autotransformer will reduce the voltage by 50%. Depending on the application, that portion of the winding used solely in the higher-voltage (lower current) portion may be wound with wire of a smaller gauge, though the entire winding is directly connected.

TRANSFORMER LOSSES

An ideal transformer generally does not have energy losses, and would be 100% efficient. But in practical transformers, energy is dissipated in the windings, core, and surrounding structures. Transformer losses are divided into load losses and no load losses.

Transformer No Load Losses

The no-load losses are essentially the power required to keep the core energized. These are commonly referred to as "core losses," and they exist whenever the unit is energized. No-load losses depend primarily upon the voltage and frequency, so under operational conditions they vary only slightly with system variations. They include losses due to magnetization of the core, dielectric losses in the insulation, and winding losses due to the flow of the exciting current and any circulating currents in parallel conductors. They include:

Eddy current losses are caused by varying magnetic fields inducing eddy currents in the laminations and thus generating heat. These losses can be reduced by building the core from thin laminated sheets insulated from each other by a thin varnish layer to reduce eddy currents.

Transformer Load Losses

Load losses, as the terminology might suggest, result from load currents flowing through the transformer. Transformer load losses include:

Ohmic heat loss, sometimes are referred as copper loss (I^2R) occurs in transformer windings and is caused by the resistance of the conductor. The magnitude of these losses increases with the square of the load current and is proportional to the resistance of the winding. Conductor eddy current losses. Eddy currents, due to magnetic fields caused by alternating current, also occur in the windings. Reducing the cross-section of the conductor reduces eddy currents.

Stray loss occurs due to the stray flux which introduces losses in the core, clamps, tank and other iron parts.

RECTIFICATION

Rectification is the process of changing alternating current into direct current and the device that produces the change is called a rectifier. Thus they allow electric current to flow in one direction but not in the other. They are incorporated into the X-ray circuit in series with the X-ray tube. Exactly the same current flows through the X-ray tube and the rectifiers.

Methods of Rectifying an Alternating Current

There are two main systems of rectification:
1. Self rectification
2. Conventional vacuum tube or solid state diode rectification.

Vacuum tube diodes also called valve tubes were used for many years in radiographic equipment. However solid state diodes have supplanted valve tubes in modern diagnostic units both single and three phase. All rectifying systems are connected between the secondary side of the X-ray transformer and the X-ray tube.

- *Self rectification*: It is the simplest type in which the high voltage is applied directly to the terminals of the X-ray tube. Under ordinary conditions, an X-ray tube allows passage of electrons from the cathode to the anode during the positive half of the cycle of the AC curve when the anode is positively charged. This half of the cycle is useful voltage or forward bias. During the negative half of the cycle no current will flow inspite of anode being negative because there is no space charge near the anode. At the same time the reverse voltage also known as the inverse voltage or reverse bias is actually higher than the useful voltage. This is caused by transformer regulation, a condition associated with power loss in the transformer core and characterized by a slight fall in kV accompanying the flow of tube current during forward bias.

- *Diode rectification:* A diode normally passes current in one direction only that is electrons flow from cathode to anode. Either one or two diodes can provide half wave rectification also known as one-pulse rectification. Electrons flow readily from the cathode to anode in one half of the cycle. During the next half of the cycle the polarity of the transformer is reversed and electrons cannot flow from anode to cathode in the rectifier diode, thereby protecting the X-ray tube from the inverse voltage, also called reverse bias. With two rectifier diodes, the high voltage during the negative half of the cycle is divided among the diodes and the X-ray tube, thereby increasing the efficiency of the system and improving the heat loading capacity of the X-ray tube. Four rectifier diodes can be arranged to provide full wave rectification.

Solid State Rectifiers

High voltage rectifiers can be of conventional vacuum – tube type (often called thermionic diode tubes) or they can be of solid state composition. These thermionic diode tubes were used in the past in the Coolidge X-ray tube. In modern equipment, conventional vacuum rectifiers are no longer used. As compared to conventional vacuum rectifiers, solid state rectifiers are smaller, more reliable and have a longer life.

Selenium was the first material used for a solid state rectifier. The heart of a solid state rectifier is a semiconductor which is usually a piece of crystalline silicon. Silicon contains four valence electrons. In a solid, such as silicon, there are numerous energy levels permissible for electrons. The valence electrons must lose or gain energy to move from one energy level to another. Electrons in the conduction band—(which corresponds to unfilled energy levels) are relatively free from atomic bonding and may move freely through the semiconductor material.

N-type semiconductors: Silicon contains four valence electrons. If a material with five valence electrons is added as an impurity to the silicon lattice, the added atoms will take the place of some silicon atoms throughout the crystal. One of the five valence electrons of the impurity is not utilized in the bonding with silicon. This unbound electron can move about in the crystal much easier than one of the bound electrons. The impurity is called a *donor* since it donates an, extra electron. The crystal resulting from the addition of the donor is called *N-type,* with N derived from the negative

charge of the surplus electron. The most commonly used donor materials are arsenic and antimony.

P-type semiconductors: If an impurity with only three valence electrons is added to silicon, the impurity atom will have only three electrons to share with four surrounding silicon atoms. One silicon atom now has an electron that is looking for another electron with which to form a covalent bond. The absence of this electron is called a "hole." Since the hole is a positive "particle," as compared to the negative electron, the material is called a *P-type* semi-conductor.

When N-type and P-type crystals are joined, a *P-N junction* is created. The N-type material is rich in electrons and the P-type is rich in holes. When the junction is formed, electrons diffuse across the junction that limits diffusion. When electrons leave the N-type material, the junction area is left with a net positive charge. Similarly, the P-type material acquires a negative charge. This creates what is called a "depletion layer." The depletion layer has a junction potential that is opposite in sign to the designation of the materials (i.e. the junction potential is positive on the side of the N-type and negative on the side of the P-type material). The device formed by a P-N junction is called a *diode. Solid-state rectifiers are diodes.*

Silicon rectifiers: A single silicon rectifier (called a cell) will resist a reverse voltage of about 1000 V, which is 10 to 20 times higher than a selenium rectifier. Silicon rectifiers can withstand a temperature of up to 392°C, considerably higher than selenium at 266°C. A silicon rectifier is made up of a number of cells, or individual diodes, connected together to form a cylindrical stack that might have dimensions of 20 to 30 cm long by 20 mm diameter. Such a rectifier can operate up to 150 kVp and 1000 mA. Modern X-ray equipment uses solid state silicon rectifiers.

Half-wave rectification: When the voltage reverses during the inverse half of the alternating cycle, the rectifier stops current flow. When rectifiers are used in this manner they produce half-wave rectification. The only advantage of the rectifiers is that they protect the X-ray tube from the full potential of the inverse cycle.

Full-wave rectification: Modern X-ray generators employ full-wave rectification, which utilizes the full potential of the electrical supply. Both halves of the alternating voltage are used to produce X-rays, so the X-ray output per unit time is twice as large as it is with half-wave rectification.

Test for Working of a Rectifier System

The simplest device for testing the competence of any type of rectifier diode is the spinning top. This is flat metal top which has a small hole punched near one edge. It is placed on a film exposure holder containing an X-ray film and made to spin during an X-ray exposure of one tenth second. If all four diodes are operating, the circuit is fully rectified and there should be 120 pulses per sec with 120 corresponding peaks of X-ray output on 60 cycles current. Therefore in one-tenth second there will be twelve peaks and the image of the spinning top on the radiograph will shows twelve spots. If only six dark spots appear in the radiograph of the top, there were only six pulses in one-tenth second or sixty pulses per second indicating that the circuit is half wave rectified.

ELECTRONIC TIMER

Timer is a mechanical or electronic device whose action is to make or break the high voltage across the X-ray tube.

In electronic timers the length of the X-ray exposure is determined by the time required to charge a capacitor through a selected resistance. The exposure button starts the exposure and also starts charging the capacitor. The exposure is terminated when the capacitor is charged to a value necessary to turn on associated electronic circuits. The exposure time is therefore determined by the length of time for the capacitor to charge, and this time can be varied by varying the value of the resistance in the charging circuit.

Electronic timers are precise and accurate. They have an important role for the Quality Assurance of medical diagnostic X-ray machines. The X-ray sensor allows direct measurement of exposure from the X-ray head. Pulses produced by half wave and full-wave X-ray are measured as 60 or 120 pulses per second. There is no need to reset the instrument after each reading. It is circuit consists of thyratron tube or thyristor. The advantages of electronic timer are it allows wide range of time intervals and allows serial exposures. Nowadays controlled by microprocessor.

COOLING OF X-RAY TUBE

Large amount of heat is generated in the operation of an X-ray which can melt the tungsten target. Various steps are developed to dissipate the heat and protect the tube. The X-ray tube uses all three forms of cooling—radiation, conduction, and convection.

An X-ray tube is enclosed within an X-ray tube housing which is a chamber filled with oil or other cooling medium for cooling the X-ray tube. The X-ray tube includes an envelope enclosing an evacuated chamber in which an anode assembly is mounted to a bearing assembly and interacts with a cathode assembly for production of X-rays. A heat sink is coupled to the bearing assembly and provides a thermally conductive path between the bearing assembly and the cooling medium in the X-ray tube housing for providing direct cooling of the bearing assembly during operation. Tube housing absorbs most of off-focus radiation and helps to cool the tube. Some housing have fan for cooling. Since the housing is generally cooled by the movement of air, or convection, its effective capacity can be increased by using forced air circulation.

Cooling of anode is important for proper functioning. Construction of the anode with two metals—one with a very high melting point (tungsten) and the other with a high conductivity for heat (copper) helps in cooling of anode.

The main cooling methods that are used or have been used are as follows:

- *Natural radiation:* In this heat is lost via the glass tube into the air.
- *Air cooling by radiation:* A radiator may be attached to the extreme end of the anode to increase the surface area which can give off heat into the air.
- *Oil cooling:* Almost all X-ray tubes in use today are surrounded by oil. The oil insulates as well as cools. Oil and air cooling may be combined.
- *The rotating anode tube:* As the name implies the anode target rotates during the exposure. This allows us to increase the exposure because of the tremendous ability to dissipate heat.

FOCAL SPOT

Focal spot is the region of an X-ray tube on the anode that is struck by electrons from which the X-rays are emitted.

The smaller the focal spot the better the resolution of the resultant image. Unfortunately, as the size of the focal spot decreases, the heat of the target is concentrated into a smaller area and can eventually be so high as to vaporize the material, leading to tube failure. This is the limiting factor to focal spot size. Many X-ray tubes have two focal spot sizes that can be selected by the operator. The small focal spot is generally used at relatively low power (kV and mA) settings. The large focal spot is used when the machine must be operated at power levels that exceed the rated capacity of the small focal spot. The effective focal spot is the beam projected onto the patient. The anode angle θ determines the effective focal spot size. As the anode angle decreases, the effective focal spot decreases. Diagnostic tube target angles range from 5° to 15°.

Measuring Focal Spot Size

Pinhole camera consists of a very small circular aperture (10 to 30 mm diameter) in a disk made of a thin, highly attenuating metal such as lead, tungsten, or gold. The image of focal spot is recorded with the pinhole camera positioned on the central axis between the X-ray source and the detector.

Slit camera: The slit camera consists of a plate made of a highly attenuating metal (often tungsten) with a thin slit (typically 10 mm wide). Measuring the width of the distribution on the image yields one dimension of the focal spot. Second radiograph, taken with the slit perpendicular to the first, yields the other dimension of the focal spot

Star pattern: Star pattern test tool contains a radial pattern of lead spokes of diminishing width and spacing on a thin plastic disk. Imaging the star pattern at a known magnification and measuring the distance between the outermost blur patterns on the image provides an estimate of the resolving power of the focal spot in the directions perpendicular to and parallel to the anode-cathode axis

Resolution bar pattern: Similar to the star pattern tool, but containing radiopaque bars of varying widths and spacings. Bar pattern images demonstrate the effective resolution parallel and perpendicular to the anode-cathode axis for a given magnification geometry.

ANODE HEEL EFFECT

X-ray beam intensity is not uniform throughout its entirety. As the anode is angled, the intensity of the X-ray beam along the longitudinal axis of the tube varies. This phenomenon consists of a reduction of X-ray intensity towards the anode side of the X-ray beam (Fig. 2.9), owing to the higher absorption of those X-rays that pass through a greater thickness of material as they emerge from the target. The fact that the intensities vary in such a manner causes visible differences in the density produced on the radiographs. This phenomenon is called heel effect.

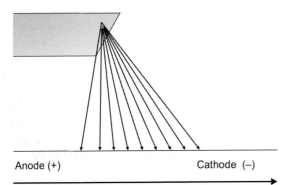

Anode (+)   Cathode (−)

Intensity in creases towards cathode side

Fig. 2.9 Heel effect shows reduction of X-ray intensity towards the anode side of the X-ray beam

In tubes with small angles, this is more pronounced and limits the size of the useful beam. Heel effect is noticeable in diagnostic radiography because of the easy absorption of low energy photons generated and because of the steep target angles used. The resulting radiograph of an object of equal density and thickness will be darker on that part of the radiograph near the cathode and lighter on that part of the radiograph near the anode. This inequality intensity can be used to the advantage of the radiographer by positioning the heavier or denser part of the patient on the end of the table under the cathode. The portion of the X-ray beam with the greatest intensity will then pass through the portion of the body with the greatest density as seen in leg. By placing the proximal end of the leg under the cathode side of the tube, the finished radiograph would have balanced density. The heel effect will be much less noticeable if the focal-film distance is large. Conversely, if the focal-film distance is shortened, the effect of the unequal intensity within the X-ray beam will be noticed more. The heel effect will be noticed more on exposing a large film as compared to a small film.

SPECTRUM OUT OF X-RAY TUBE

Spectrum coming out of X-ray tube consists of a X-Ray photons which are electromagnetic radiation with wavelengths in the range 0.1 to 100 Å. Electromagnetic radiation is made up of waves of energy that contain electric and magnetic fields vibrating transversely and sinusoidally to each other and to the direction of propagation of the waves.

X-rays are generated by two different processes, resulting in the production of a continuous spectrum of X-rays. One involves reaction of the electrons with the nucleus of the tungsten atoms, producing X-rays that are termed general radiation, or bremsstrahlung. The second involves collision between the high speed electrons and the electrons in the shell of the target tungsten atoms, producing X-rays that are called characteristic radiation. The wavelength of X-rays in the spectrum varies.

The quantity (number) of the X-rays generated is proportional to the atomic number of the target material (Z), the square of the kilovoltage (kVp^2), and the milliamperes of X-ray tube current (mA). The quality (energy) of the X-rays generated depends almost entirely on the X-ray tube potential (kVp).

Filtration is the process of shaping the X-ray beam to increase the ratio of photons useful for imaging to those photons that increase patient dose or decrease image contrast. Diagnostic X-ray beams are composed of photons that have a whole spectrum of energies. They are polychromatic. As polychromatic radiation passes through a patient, most of the lower energy photons are absorbed in the first few centimeters of tissue, and only the higher energy photons penetrate through the patient to form the radiographic image. Filters are sheets of metal placed in the path of the X-ray beam near the X-ray tube housing to absorb low energy radiation before it reaches the patient. Their main function is to protect the patient from useless radiation. Aluminum is usually selected as the filter material for diagnostic radiology.

An X-ray beam restrictor is a device that is attached to the opening in the X-ray tube housing to regulate the size and shape of an X-ray beam. There are three types of X-ray beam restrictors: aperture diaphragms, cones (cylinders), and collimators. Their basic function is to regulate the size and shape of the X-ray beam. Closely collimated beams have two advantages over larger beams. First, a smaller area of the patient is exposed and, because area is a square function, a decrease of one half in X-ray beam diameter effects a fourfold decrease in patient exposure. Second, well-collimated beams generate less scatter radiation and thus improve film quality.

There are five basic ways that an X-ray photon can interact with matter. These are:
1. Coherent scattering
2. Photoelectric effect
3. Compton scattering
4. Pair production
5. Photodisintegration.

Only two interactions are important in diagnostic radiology, the photoelectric effect and Compton scattering. Coherent scattering is numerically unimportant, and pair production and photodisintegration occur at energies above the useful energy range. The photoelectric effect is the predominant interaction with low energy radiation and with high atomic number absorbers. It generates no significant scatter radiation and produces high contrast in the X-ray image but, unfortunately, exposes the patient to a great deal of radiation. At higher diagnostic energies, Compton scattering is the most common interaction between X-rays and body tissues, and is responsible for almost all scatter radiation. Radiographic image contrast is less with Compton reactions than with the photoelectric effect.

Attenuation is the reduction in the intensity of an X-ray beam as it traverses matter either by the absorption or deflection of photons from the beam. The attenuation of monochromatic radiation is exponential; that is, each layer of absorber attenuates the same percentage of the photons remaining in the beam. The attenuation of polychromatic radiation is not exponential. A large percentage of the low energy photons are attenuated by the first few centimeters of absorber, so the quality (mean energy) of the remaining photons increases as the beam passes through an absorber. The amount of attenuation depends on the energy of the radiation and three characteristics of the tissue: atomic number, density, and electrons per gram. Increasing the radiation energy increases the number of transmitted photons, while increasing the atomic number, density, or electrons per gram decreases transmission. Energy and atomic number together determine the relative percentage of photoelectric and Compton reactions. With low energy radiation, and with high atomic number absorbers, a large amount of photoelectric attenuation is superimposed on a small background of Compton attenuation. As the energy of the radiation is increased, photoelectric attenuation diminishes, until the background of Compton attenuation is all that remains. Density is one of the most important factors affecting attenuation, and radiographic image contrast is largely dependent on differences in tissue density. The high contrast between air and soft tissues occurs entirely because of density differences. The number of electrons per gram plays a lesser role. Generally, as the atomic number increases, the number of electrons per gram decreases, but the decrease is more than compensated by an even greater increase in density. Thus, high atomic number elements attenuate more radiation, even though they have fewer electrons per gram. The amount of scatter radiation reaching an X-ray film increases with increasing field size, part thickness, and kilovoltage.

3

X-ray Interactions

Aditi Dongre

There are five basic ways that an X-ray photon can interact with matter:
1. Coherent scattering
2. Photoelectric effect
3. Compton scattering
4. Pair production
5. Photodisintegration.

RELATIVE IMPORTANCE OF PHOTON INTERACTION TO RADIOGRAPHY

A radiograph is produced when an X-ray beam is incident on a specific part of a patient's body. As the X-ray beam enters the tissue many photons are transmitted and interact with the film causing the film to darken. When photons are absorbed they are completely removed from the X-ray beam and cease to exist.

1. *Coherent scattering:* When a low energy X-ray photon interacts with a relatively bound orbital electron, it sets the electron into vibration. This produces an electromagnetic wave identical in energy to that of the incident photon but differing in direction. Thus in effect the entering photon has been scattered without undergoing any change in wavelength, frequency or energy but differing in direction. There are two types of coherent scattering, Thomson scattering and Rayleigh scattering. In Thomson scattering a single electron is involved in the interaction. Rayleigh scattering results from the co-operative interaction with all the electrons of an atom. In coherent scattering there is no transfer of energy and no ionization occurs.

2. *Photoelectric effect:* Simply stated, the photoelectric effect occurs when photons interact with matter with resulting ejection of electrons from the matter. It occurs when the energy of the incident photon is slightly greater than the binding energy of the electrons in one of the inner shells. Photoelectric (PE) absorption of X-rays occurs when the X-ray photon is absorbed resulting in the ejection of electrons from the inner shell (K-shell) of the

atom. The atom is left with an electron void in the K-shell but only for an instant. The electron usually comes from the adjacent L-shell occasionally from the M-shell and on rare occasions from the same or another atom. This leaves the atom in an ionized state. The ionized atom then returns to the neutral state with the emission of an X-ray characteristic of the atom (Fig. 3.1). PE absorption is the dominant process for X-ray absorption up to energies of about 500 KeV (Fig. 3.2). PE absorption is also dominant for atoms of high atomic numbers. The photoelectric effect is responsible for the production of characteristic X-rays in the X-ray tube, but the process is also important as a secondary process that occurs when X-rays interact with matter. An X-ray photon transfers its energy to an orbital electron, which is then dislodged and

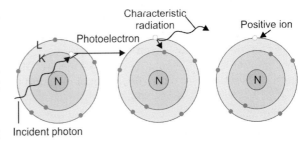

Fig. 3.1 Photoelectric effect

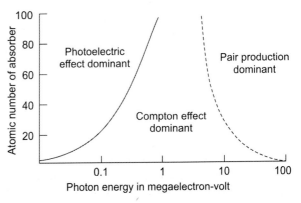

Fig. 3.2 X-ray interaction with absorber on the basis of energy of photon and atomic number of absorber

exits the atom at high speed with a kinetic energy equal to:

$$KE = E - P$$

Where, KE is the kinetic energy of the photoelectron, E is the energy of the incident X-ray photon. P is the energy required to remove the electron. This is equivalent to its binding energy in the atom.

APPLICATIONS OF PHOTOELECTRIC EFFECT IN DIAGNOSTIC RADIATION

The photoelectric effect gives two types of radiation, photoelectrons and characteristic X-rays. The photoelectric effect is very important in radiography because the chance of its occurrence varies directly with the atomic number of the irradiated tissue and indirectly with the photon energy.

Basically it produces radiographic images of excellent quality. The quality is good for two reasons: first the photoelectric effect does not produce scatter radiation and second it enhances natural tissue contrast. So from the point of view of the film quality, photoelectric effect is desirable while from the point of view of the patient exposure it is undesirable because patients receive more radiation.

The Compton Effect or Compton scattering (C), also known an incoherent scattering, occurs when the incident X-ray photon ejects an electron from an atom and an X-ray photon of lower energy is scattered from the atom. Relativistic energy and momentum are conserved in this process and the scattered X-ray photon has less energy and therefore greater wavelength than the incident photon. Compton Scattering is important for low atomic number specimens. At energies of 100 keV to 10 MeV (Fig. 3.1) the absorption of radiation is mainly due to the Compton Effect.

The Compton Effect will occur with very low atomic weight targets even at relatively low X-ray energies. The effect may be thought of as a scattering of the photons by atomic electrons. In the process, also called Compton scattering, the incident X-ray changes direction and loses energy, imparting that energy to the electron (now called a Compton electron or recoil electron). This phenomenon was discovered by renowned physicist, A. H. Compton. The emerging photon, having undergone a change in direction is called a scattered photon.

Scatter radiation: It refers to those X-ray photons that have undergone a change in direction after interacting with atoms. The primary X-ray beam leaving the X-ray tube is polyenergetic, i.e. it contains photons of various energies. As the primary beam passes through the patient some of the radiation is absorbed while the rest is scattered in many directions. In the diagnostic range the scattered radiation generated in the body consists mainly of scattered photons produced by Compton scattering, but also includes characteristic radiation resulting from photoelectric interaction. The multidirectional scattered radiation is a noise factor which seriously impairs radiographic quality by its fogging effect diffusing X rays over the surface of the film and thereby lessening the contrast. Radiographic image contrast is less with compton reactions than with the photoelectric effect.

Factors affecting scatter radiation: Scatter radiation is maximum with high kvp techniques, large fields and thick parts. Three factors determine the quantity of scatter radiation. These are: Field size; Part thickness and Kilovoltage.

- *Field size* is the most important factor in the production of scatter radiation. A small X-ray field (usually called a narrow beam) irradiates only a small amount of tissues so it generates only a small amount of scattered photons. A large X-ray field is enlarged; the quantity of scatter radiation increases rapidly at first and finally tapers off and reaches a plateau.

- *Part thickness:* The number of scattered photons increases with increase in the part thickness. It is difficult to control this factor as patients are of different thickness.

- *Kilovoltage:* The effect of kilovoltage is not as important as field size and part thickness. In low energy range (20 to 30 keV) in which the photoelectric effect predominates, extremely little scatter radiation is produced. As the radiation energy increases the percentage of Compton reaction increases so does the production of scatter radiation.

- *Pair production:* It does not occur in diagnostic energy range. In this process a high energy (Fig. 3.1) photon (1.02 MeV) interacts with the nucleus of an atom, the photon disappears and its energy converted into matter in the form of two particles. One is an ordinary electron and the other is a positron, a particle with the same mass as an electron but with a positive charge.

- *Photo disintegration:* In this process part of the nucleus of an atom is ejected by a high energy photon. The ejected portion may be a neutron, a proton, an alpha particle or cluster of particles. The photon should have sufficient energy to overcome nuclear binding energies of the order of 7 to 15 MeV.

ATTENUATION

Attenuation is defined as the process of removal of photons from an X-ray beam as it passes through an absorber which results from photoelectric absorption, compton scattering, pair production or photo disintegration.

The attenuation of monochromatic radiation is exponential that is each layer of absorber attenuates the same percentage of the photons remaining in the beam. The attenuation of polychromatic radiation is not exponential. A large percentage of the low energy photons are attenuated by the first few centimeters of the absorber so the quality of the remaining photons increases as the beam passes through an absorber.

As a photon makes its way through matter, there is no way to predict precisely either how far it will travel before engaging in an interaction or the type of interaction it will engage in. In clinical applications we are generally not concerned with the fate of an individual photon but rather with the collective interaction of the large number of photons. In most instances we are interested in the overall rate at which photons interact as they make their way through a specific material.

Attenuation coefficient: An attenuation coefficient is a measure of the quantity of radiation attenuated by a given thickness of an absorber. Two are important in diagnostic radiology; linear and mass attenuation coefficient.

Let us observe what happens when a group of photons encounters a slice of material that is 1 unit thick, as illustrated in the Figure 3.3. Some of the photons interact with the material, and some pass on through. The interactions, either photoelectric or Compton, remove some of the photons from the beam in a process known as attenuation. Under specific conditions, a certain percentage of the photons will interact, or be attenuated, in a 1-unit thickness of material.

Linear attenuation coefficient (Fig. 3.3): The linear attenuation coefficient (μ) is the actual fraction of photons interacting per 1-unit thickness of material. In our example the fraction that interacts in the 1 cm thickness is 0.1, or 10%, and the value of the linear attenuation coefficient is 0.1 per cm. Linear attenuation coefficient values indicate the rate at which photons interact as they move through material and are inversely related to the average distance photons travel before interacting. The rate at which photons interact (attenuation coefficient value) is determined by the energy of the individual photons and the atomic number and density of the material.

Mass attenuation coefficient: In some situations it is more desirable to express the attenuation rate in terms of the mass of the material encountered by the photons rather than in terms of distance (Fig. 3.4). The quantity that affects attenuation rate is not the total mass of an object but rather the area mass. Area mass is the amount of material behind a 1-unit surface area, as shown below. The area mass is the product of material thickness and density:

Area Mass (g/cm^2) =
Thickness (cm) × Density (g/cm^3)

The mass attenuation coefficient is the rate of photon interactions per 1-unit (g/cm^2) area mass.

The figure compares two pieces of material with different thicknesses and densities but the same area mass. Since both attenuate the same fraction of photons, the mass attenuation coefficient is the same for the two materials. They do not have the same linear attenuation coefficient values.

The relationship between the mass and linear attenuation coefficients is

Mass Attenuation Coefficient (μ/ρ) =
Linear Attenuation Coefficient (μ)/Density (ρ).

The symbol for mass attenuation coefficient (μ/ρ) is derived from the symbols for the linear attenuation coefficient (μ) and the symbol for density (ρ). We must be careful not to be misled by the relationship stated in this manner. Confusion often arises as to the effect of material density on attenuation coefficient values. Mass attenuation coefficient values are actually normalized with respect to material density, and therefore do not change with changes in density. Material density does

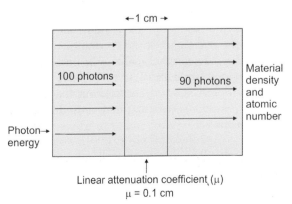

Fig. 3.3 Linear attenuation coefficient depends on material density, atomic number and photon energy

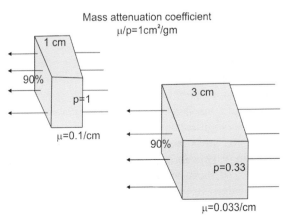

Fig. 3.4 Mass attenuation coefficient

have a direct effect on linear attenuation coefficient values.

The total attenuation rate depends on the individual rates associated with photoelectric and Compton interactions. The respective attenuation coefficients are related as follows:

$$\mu_{(total)} = \mu_{(photoelectric)} + \mu_{(Compton)}$$

Factors affecting attenuation: Factors determine the degree of attenuation of an X-ray beam as it passes through matter include the nature of the radiation and the composition of matter. Increasing the radiation energy increases the number of transmitted photons while increasing the density, atomic number or electrons per gram of the absorber decreases the number of transmitted photons.

Applications to Diagnostic Radiology

- The transmitted and attenuated photons are equally important. If all photons were transmitted the film would be uniformly black; if all photons were attenuated then film would be uniformly white. In neither case would there be an X-ray image. Image formation depends on a differential attenuation between tissues.
- The higher the linear attenuation coefficient, the greater the attenuation. Therefore X-ray attenuation is greater in bone than in water.
- At low photon energies most of the difference in X-ray attenuation between bone and soft tissues results from a difference in the number of photoelectric reaction while at high photon energies the difference in X-ray attenuation between bone and soft tissues is almost entirely the result of the difference in the number of Compton reactions.

SCATTERED RADIATION

Scatter radiations arise from interactions of the primary radiation beam with the atoms in the object being imaged. When X-ray radiation passes through a patient, three types of interactions can occur, including coherent scattering (coherent scatter), photoelectric absorption and Compton scattering. Of these three events, the great majority of scattered X-rays in diagnostic X-ray imaging arise from Compton scattering. Because the scattered radiation deviates from the straight line path between the X-ray focus and the image receptor, scattered radiation is a major source of image degradation. This scattered radiation reduces image contrast. The degree of contrast loss depends on the scatter content of the radiation emerging from the patient's body. Scattered radiation is a noise factor which seriously impairs radiographic quality by its fogging effect and lessening contrast.

Techniques to Minimize Scattered Radiation

Collimation: The amount of scattered radiation is generally proportional to the total primary X-ray beam. This is, in turn, determined by the thickness of the patient and the area or field size being exposed. Increasing the field size increases the total amount of scattered radiation and the value of the scatter contrast-reduction factors. Therefore, one method of reducing scattered radiation and increasing contrast is to reduce the field size with X-ray beam collimators, cones, or other beam-limiting devices. Contrast can be improved by reducing the field size to the smallest practical value in some situation.

Air gap: The quantity of scattered radiation in an X-ray beam reaching a receptor can be reduced by separating the patient's body and receptor surface. This separation is known as an air gap. Scattered radiation leaving a patient's body is more divergent than the primary X-ray beam. The reduction of scattered radiation in proportion to primary radiation increases with air-gap distance. Patient exposure is increased because of the inverse-square effect. The use of an air gap introduces magnification. Therefore, a larger receptor size is required to obtain the same patient area coverage. If the air gap is obtained by increasing the tube-to-receptor distance, the X-ray equipment must be operated at a higher output to obtain adequate receptor exposure.

Grid: The most effective and practical method of removing a portion of the scattered radiation is to use a grid. The grid is placed between the patient's body and the receptor. It is constructed of alternate strips of an X-ray-absorbing material, such as lead, and a relatively nonabsorbing interspace material, such as fiber, carbon, or aluminum. The grid strips are aligned with the direction of the primary X-ray beam. The focal point of the grid should coincide with the focal spot of the X-ray tube. Because the X-ray beam direction is aligned with the grid, much of the primary radiation passes through the interspaces without encountering the lead strips. Since scattered radiation is not generally lined up with the grid strips, a large portion of it is absorbed by the grid. The ideal grid would absorb all scattered radiation and allow all primary X-rays to penetrate to the receptor.

4
Grids, Collimators, Filters

Rajlaxmi Sharma

X-rays have been integral part of diagnostic radiology since their discovery in 1895. As discussed earlier X-ray beams are polychromatic and contain X-ray photons of different energies and wavelengths. The useful energy range in radiography is about 25 to 120 kVp. The low kVp X-ray beams are not useful for radiograph development as they get absorbed at the superficial part of tissue. Therefore, it is better to filter them before they reach the patient.

The nature of X-ray beams and their reactions with the tissue have already been discussed in previous chapters. As the primary X-ray beam passes through the object, some of the radiation is absorbed and rest is scattered in different directions. In diagnostic radiology, most of the scattered radiation is produced by compton effect with some contribution by characteristic radiation resulting from photoelectric effect. These scattered radiations seriously degrade the radiographic quality and also increases patient radiation dose. Certain devices are required for modifying X-ray beam and restricting non required X-rays to decrease radiation exposure to patient and to improve radiographic quality by improving contrast and clarity.

GRIDS

Scattered radiation cannot be entirely eliminated, it can be reduced with special devices to improve radiographic quality. Most effective in minimizing radiation scatter are the stationary grid and the moving grid.

Stationary Grid

Invented by Dr Gustave Bucky in 1913, stationary grid is the most effective method to get rid of scattered radiations from radiographic field. It is placed between the patient and the cassette. The original grid developed by Bucky was cross hatch type with wide lead strips arranged in parallel and perpendicular to this parallel series. Even though scattered radiation was significantly reduced grid pattern used to appear on the radiograph.

The modern radiographic grids consist of series of lead foil strips separated by X-ray transparent spaces. The interspaces of grids are filled either with aluminum or other organic component. It supports the thin lead foil stripes. The lead foil absorbs most of scatter radiation and the interspaces allow primary radiation to reach the cassette. Nowadays these are built into the cassette front called as grid cassette. As exposure factors needs to be increased while using grids, intensifying screens must be used with them.

Factors determining grids ability to improve contrast are its lead content, grid ratio and grid frequency.

- *Lead content of grid:* The amount of lead in a grid is a good indicator of its ability to improve contrast. It is measured as mass per unit area in g/cm^2 of the grid surface. For example a grid with thicker strips is more efficient in reducing scattered radiation; however, it will also remove more primary radiation necessitating larger exposure.

- *Grid ratio:* Grid ratio is defined as ratio between the height of the lead strips and distance between the lead strips. Thus Grid ratio is determined by dividing the height of the radiopaque strip (h) by the width of the interspace material (D), giving equation: grid ratio = h/D. Grid ratio is expressed in two numbers and usually varies between 4:1 to 16:1. Grid ratio determines the ability of grid to remove scatter radiation; higher the ratio, better the grid function.

- *Grid frequency/Lines per inch:* It is the number of lead strips per inch or per cm of grid.

   Grid frequency/lines/inch = 25.4/D + d

   Where,
   25.4 – The number of mm per inch
   D – Thickness of interspaces
   d – Thickness of lead strips

- *Grid pattern:* It is the pattern of grid that we see from top view to see the orientation of lead strips in their longitudinal axis.

   - *Linear grid:* In the linear grid, the lead strips are parallel to each other in their longitudinal axis (Fig. 4.1). These are mainly used in

Fig. 4.1 Linear grid has lead strips only in one direction

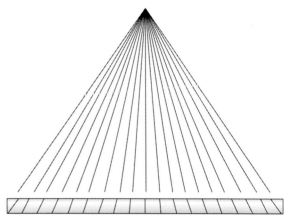

Fig. 4.3 Focused linear grid

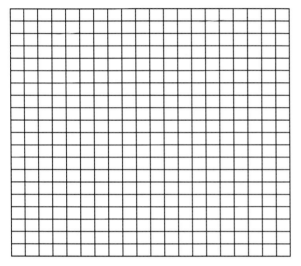

Fig. 4.2 Crossed grid

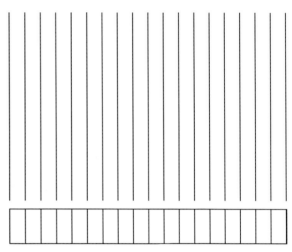

Fig. 4.4 Parallel grid: Infinite focal distance

fluoroscopy. It allows us to angle the X-ray tube along the length of the grid without loss of primary radiation from grid cut off centrally. However, it has high peripheral cut off causing progressively more absorption of X-ray towards the sides of the grid relative to the center.

– *Crossed grid:* Crossed grid is made of two superimposed linear grids that have the same focusing distance (Fig. 4.2). It consists of two sets of grid lines arranged perpendicular to each other. Grid ratio of crossed grids is equal to the sum of the ratio of the two linear grids. These grids cannot be used with oblique techniques requiring angulation of X-ray tube and have limited use in general radiology because of the excessive cut off.

– *Focused grid:* This is a grid made up of lead strips that are angled slightly so that they focus

in space (Fig. 4.3). Focused grids could be linear or crossed grids. Linear grids have convergent line and crossed grids have convergent point. Focal distance is the perpendicular distance between the grid and convergent line or point. Focusing range is the distance within which grid can be used. Low ratio grids have wide focusing range, while high ratio grids have narrow focusing range.

• *Parallel grid:* Parallel grid is the one in which the lead strips are parallel when viewed in cross section. They are focused at infinity and are generally used with small X-ray fields like fluoroscopy spot film devices (Fig. 4.4).

Evaluation of Grid Performance

An ideal grid should absorb all secondary radiation and no primary radiation to improve contrast of film and reduce patient exposure. But such grid does not exist. We have to weigh these two factors in clinical practice to evaluation grid performance. There are three methods of evaluating grid performance.

1. *Primary transmission:* Primary transmission is a measurement of primary radiation transmitted through grid. Ideally grid should transmit 100% of primary radiation as it creates the radiographic image. However, in practice there is significant loss of primary radiation with grids. The measured primary transmission is always less than the calculated primary transmission.

2. *Bucky or grid factor (B):* The Bucky factor is the ratio of the incident radiation falling on the grid to the transmitted radiation passing through the grid.

B = Incident radiation/Transmitted radiation

As Bucky factor measure the total quantity of radiation absorbed from an X-ray beam by a grid, it measures grids ability to absorb scattered radiation. The Bucky factor is measured by giving trial exposures with a phantom. Higher the Bucky factor, more is the scatter radiation absorption and lower the Bucky factor, lesser the scatter radiation absorption. However, higher Bucky factor is associated with greater radiation dosage to patient.

3. *Contrast improvement factor:* The contrast improvement factor (K) is the ratio of the contrast with a grid to the contrast without a grid.

K = Contrast with grid/Contrast without grid

The contrast improvement factor is the ultimate test of the grid performance as it measures the grid's ability to improve contrast which is its primary function. However, it is affected by kVp, field size and phantom thickness.

Grid cut off: The Grid cut off is defined as loss of primary radiation due to use of grid. There are two major disadvantage of use of grid. Foremost is the increased radiation dose to patient. They also require proper centering of X-ray tube, otherwise may lead to loss of primary radiation which carries important information. Grid cut off occurs due to poor geometric relationship between the primary beam and lead foil strips of the grid. Cutoff is complete and no primary radiation reaches the film when the projected images of the lead strips are thicker than the width of interspaces. The film so produced will have less density or will be light in the area in which cut off occurs. There are four situations that produce grid cutoff.

1. *Focused grids used upside down:* Focused grids have the tube side which indicates the focus of lead strips. When it is used upside down there is severe

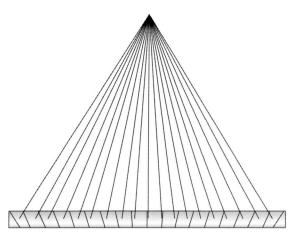

Fig. 4.5 Grid cut-off with use of an inverted grid

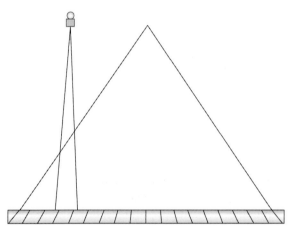

Fig. 4.6 Grid cut-off with use of a laterally centered tube

peripheral cut off with dark band of exposure in the centre of the film (Fig. 4.5).

2. *Lateral decentering:* Lateral decentering results from the X-ray tube being positioned lateral to the convergent line but at the correct focal distance. All the lead strips cut off the same amount of primary radiation so there is uniform loss of radiation over the entire surface of grid producing of uniformly light radiograph (Fig. 4.6).

There are three factors which determine the cut off due to lateral decentering: (a) Grid ratio, (b) Focal distance, (c) Amount of decentering.

L = rb/fo × 100

where,
L – Loss of primary radiation (%)
r – Grid ratio
b – Lateral decentering (inches)
fo – focal distance of grids (inches)

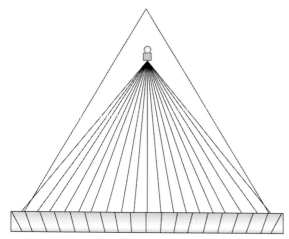

Fig. 4.7 Focused grid used at other than the correct focal-grid distance

Thus, the cut off increases as the grid ratio and decentering distance increases while cut off decreases as the focal distance increases. The lateral decentering can be minimized by use of low grid ratio and larger focal distances.

3. *Focus grid distance decentering:* If the target of X-ray tube is correctly centered to the grid, but positioned above or below the convergent line of the grid, the result is focus-grid decentering (Fig. 4.7). If the target is above the convergent line, it is called as far focus grid distance decentering and if the target is below the convergent line, it is called near focus grid distance decentering. The cutoff is more with near than with far focus grid distance decentering.

4. *Combined lateral and focus grid distance decentering:* This is the most commonly recognized cut off. It causes uneven exposure resulting in a film that is light on the one side and dark on other side. There are two types of combined decentering with tube target above the convergent line and tube target below the convergent line. The amount of cut off is directly proportional to the grid ratio and distance of decentering and has inverse relation to the focal distance.

Moving Grids

Moving grids were invented by Dr Hollis E Potter in 1920 and was called a Potter—Bucky grid, later on shortened as Bucky grid. Moving grids continuously move 1 to 3 cm back and forth throughout the exposure to blur out the shadows cast by the lead strips. They start moving when the anode begins to rotate. The grid should move parallel to the surface and also perpendicular to the long axis of lead strips. The moving grid is of focused type with thicker lead strips as its motion during the exposure blurs the grid lines on the radiograph. However, the disadvantage includes cost, subject to failure and vibration of X-ray tube. It also puts a limit on minimum exposure time and increases the patient's radiation dose.

Air Gap Techniques

It is alternate method to reduce patient exposure and improve film contrast by reducing scatter radiation reaching the film. The air gap technique is used in chest radiography and magnification radiography. Due to air gap most of scattered photons miss the film. It is effective in removing scatter radiations when scatter photons are close to the film. Larger the air gap more is the removal of scatter radiation. Optimum gap width is determined from following factors. If the part is thicker, the larger gap is more advantageous. The first inch of air gap improves contrast more than subsequent inches. Image sharpness deteriorates with increasing gap width unless the focus film distance is increased to compensate for the greater magnification. Patient exposures are usually less with air gap and magnification can be achieved without deteriorating sharpness by air gap technique.

FILTERS

Filtration is the process of shaping the X-ray beam to increase the ratio of photons useful for imaging to those photons that increase patient dose or decrease image contrast.

Principle behind use of filters: X-ray beams are polychromatic, i.e. they are composed of photons having spectrum of energies. When X-ray beam passes through patient, lower energy photons are absorbed in first few centimeter of tissue and only the higher energy photons travel through to produce radiographic image. Patient radiation dose depends on number of photons absorbed, but the photons absorbed in first few centimeters gives unnecessary radiation dose. This tissue can be protected by absorbing lower energy photons from the beam before they reach the patient by interposing filter between the patient and X-ray tube.

Types of Filtration

- *Coherent filtration:* Achieved in tube and its housing
- *Added filtration:* Sheets of metal are placed in the path of X-ray beam
- *Total filtration:* Total filtration is the sum of the inherent and added filtration.

Table 4.1 Materials responsible for inherent filtration by Trout, in 1963

Absorber	Thickness (mm)	Aluminum Equivalents (mm)
Glass envelope	1.4	0.78
Insulating oil	2.36	0.07
Bakelite window	1.02	0.05
Total	—	0.90

Table 4.2 Thickness of filters used in diagnostic radiology

Below 50 kVp	0.5 mm aluminum
50–70 kVp	1.5 mm aluminum
70 kVp and above	2.5 mm aluminum

Inherent filtration: The filtration resulting from the absorption of X-rays as they pass through the X-ray tube and its housing is called inherent filtration Materials for inherent filtration are glass envelope of X-ray tube, cooling insulating oil and X-ray window in the tube housing (Table 4.1). It is measured in aluminum or copper equivalent thickness and should vary between 0.5 to 1 mm. Disadvantage of inherent filtration is that it may lead to loss of contrast. To overcome this problem in few situations beryllium window tubes can be used.

Added filtration: Added filtration is achieved by placing absorber that is sheet of metal in the path of X-ray beam. Ideally material used for filtration should absorb all low energy photon and allow to pass all high energy photon. Unfortunately such material does not exist. Aluminum with atomic number 13 is excellent filter for low energy radiation while copper with atomic number 29 is better for high energy radiation. However copper is always used in combination with aluminum as a compound filter, where copper faces the X-ray tube and aluminum faces the patient.

Effects of Filtration

Average beam energy/penetrability depends on kVp and amount of total filtration in the beam. kVp also determines the minimum wavelength of the beam. Filtration determines the maximum wavelength of the beam Increasing either kVp or filtration will increase the average energy of the beam, allowing it to be more penetrating and of higher quality. Beam quality is measured by its half-value layer (HVL) that is thickness of a specified material (usually a metal) which reduces the exposure rate to one-half its initial value It is the most common method to measure radiation quality, i.e. penetrating power.

Filter thickness: A filter with 2 mm thickness absorbs all low energy photons less than 20 kev and is mostly sufficient for routine diagnostic radiography. The maximum thickness of filter used for diagnostic radiology is 3 mm. The national council on radiation protection and measurements has recommended the following total filtration for diagnostic radiology (Table 4.2).

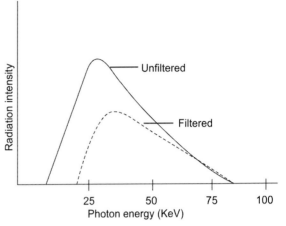

Fig. 4.8 Effect of filtration on X-ray beam

- *Effect of filtration on X-ray beam:* It increases the mean energy of X-ray beam by selectively removing the large number of low energy photons (Fig. 4.8).
- *Effect of filtration on patient exposure:* The patient exposure is remarkably reduced by use of filtration.
- *Effect of filtration exposure factors:* Filtration may lead to reduction in intensity of X-ray beam as they absorb photons at all energy levels. This is a major disadvantage and needs to be compensated by increasing exposure factors (mAs).

SPECIAL TYPES OF FILTERS

- *Wedge filters:* They are occasionally used in non uniform body parts to obtain more uniform density when part being exposed varies in thickness. The filters are wedge shaped when one side of patient is considerably thicker than the other, the wedge compensates for the difference. Less radiation is absorbed by the thinner part of the filter so more X-ray energy is available to penetrate the thicker part of patient (Fig. 4.9).
- *Heavy metal filters:* The heavy metal filters produce X-ray beam that has a high number of photons in the specific energy range which is useful in contrast imaging. Elements with atomic numbers greater than with K absorption edge close to the K-edge of the contrast are used. For example use of Gadolinium filters in iodine or barium study. The heavy metal filters transmit much narrower spectrum of X-ray energies than aluminum filter with reduction in low energy photons decrease

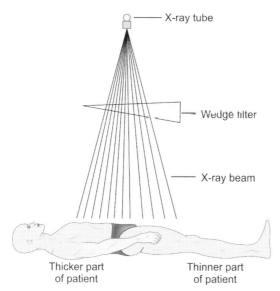

Fig. 4.9 Wedge filter

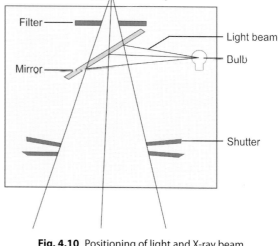

Fig. 4.10 Positioning of light and X-ray beam

the patient radiation dose and less high energy photons improves the image contrast.

• *Molybdenum filters:* Molybdenum filters are the k-edge heavy metal filters used along with molybdenum X-ray tube for mammography. Molybdenum filter of 0.30 mm thickness is used to reduce the higher energy radiation. This provides beam of upto 20 KVP thus improving the soft tissue contrast by filtering higher energy X-ray photons.

BEAM RESTRICTOR: COLLIMATORS

Collimators are best beam restrictors as it provides an infinite variety of rectangular X-ray fields and a light beam shows the center and the exact configuration of the X-ray field. They move together as a unit so that the second shutter aligns with the first to "clean up" its penumbra. The shutters functions as two adjustable aperture diaphragms. Each shutter consists of four or more lead plates. These plates move in independent pairs. One pair can be adjusted without moving the other which permits infinite variety of square or rectangular fields. When the shutters are closed they meet at the center of the X-ray field. The X-ray field is illuminated by a light beam from a light bulb in the collimator. The light beam is deflected by the mirror mounted in the path of X-ray beam at an angle of 45°. The light beam also shows the center and exact configuration of X-ray beam (Fig. 4.10).

The target of X-ray tube and light bulb should be exactly equidistant from the center of mirror so that as the light beam passes through second shutter it is collimated with X-ray beam.

Collimator helps modifying X-ray fields to desired size reducing the patient exposure. For example if 20

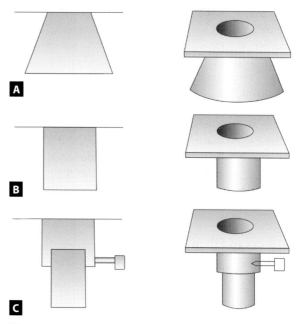

Figs 4.11A to C Beam restrictors. (A) Cone; (B) Nonadjustable cylinder; (C) Adjustable cylinder

× 20 cm field is collimated to 10 × 10 cm, the area of patient irradiated decreases from 400 cm^2 to 100 cm^2 with resultant fourfold decrease in irradiated volume. The collimators also reduce the scatter radiation. The quantity of scatter radiation reaching the X-ray film depends on field size. Smaller the field size lesser the scatter radiation and large the field size more is the scatter radiation reaching the film.

Automatic collimators are called as positive beam limiting devices. Shutters of these collimators are motor driven. When the cassette is loaded into the film holder (Bucky tray) sensor in the tray identify the size and alignment of the cassette. These sensors relay this information to the collimator motors which position the shutters to exactly match the size of the film being used.

Other Types of X-ray beam restrictors are devices which can be attached to the opening in tube housing to regulate the size and shape of X-ray beam include aperture diaphragm, cones and cylinders (Figs 4.11A to C) to decrease scatter radiation and get better films with smaller fields.

Aperture diaphragms are sheet of lead with a hole in the center are simple type of restrictors. The size and shape of the hole will determine the size and shape of the X-ray beam. Large penumbra at the periphery of the X-ray beam is the disadvantage. The width of the penumbra can be reduced by placing the aperture diaphragm as far as possible from the X-ray target.

Cones are less effective as the flare of the cone is greater than the flare of X-ray beam. Cylinders are more effective as beam restriction takes place at the far end of the barrel, so there is less penumbra. Major disadvantage of aperture diaphragms, cones and cylinder is they limit field sizes.

5

X-ray Films

Subodh Laul

The *daguerreotype* was the first commercially successful photographic process. The image was a direct positive made in the camera on a light-sensitive (by means of chemicals) surface of silver plated copper plate and did not use film at all. Starting in 1850s, thin glass plates coated with photographic emulsion became the standard medium. The flexible photographic roll film was marketed in 1885. Until 1933 X-ray films were in the form of thin glass plates coated with photographic emulsion. It was only after 1933 that flexible X-ray films were commercially made available.

TYPES OF X-RAY FILMS

- *Direct exposure film:* These types of films are used without intensifying screens and have a thicker emulsion base than screen film type. It is not used nowadays.
- *Screen film:* It is the most commonly used type of film. The film is sensitized to the light color emitted by the screen. It has improved speed and quality of radiograph.
- *Mammography film:* It is a single coated film to be used with single screen. It is made fast enough to reduce the radiation dose to breast tissue.
- *Duplicating film:* It is often necessary to send a copy of films to another specialist, or to obtain a preauthorization from the insurance company. In order to get this copy, the film needs to be duplicated. A duplicate film is made by directing a light source through the original film onto special duplicating film. The original film must be in tight contact with the duplicating film. This is accomplished by closing the lid on the duplicator and locking it or pushing down on it. Duplicating film has a single emulsion layer. The emulsion side must be in contact with the original film. Duplicating film is a direct positive film, meaning that it gives a positive, or duplicate, image of the original film. If you increase the amount of time the light is on, the duplicate film will be lighter; less light exposure creates a darker duplicate film.

The two basic components of a film are:

1. *Base:* It consists of a transparent sheet of polyster plastic which is about 0. 2 mm thick and is usually tinted blue. Modern X-ray films are called safety films because there is no flammable substance in them.
2. *Emulsion:* It consists of crystals of silver halide suspended in gelatin. The silver halide mainly consists of silver bromide and a small amount of silver iodide.

The gelatin is obtained mainly from cattle skins and bones treated with mustard oil which provides traces of sulfur and thus increases sensitivity of film. Gelatin is dissolved in hot water to which are added silver nitrate and potassium bromide in absolute darkness to produce silver bromide and silver iodide. The mixture is then heated to 50–80°C to improve the sensitivity of emulsion. This process is called digestion. It is then cooled, shredded, washed and mixed with additional gelatin. Gelatin keeps the emulsion permeable to action by processing chemicals and keeps the silver halides uniformly dispersed in the emulsion.

The emulsion is spread on polyster base to which an adhesive is attached. The layer of emulsion is about 0. 2 mm thick. The emulsion is applied to both sides of the base. Such films are called double coated films. Single coated films in which emulsion is applied to only one side are used in mammography. It must be known that the entire process must be carried out in total darkness.

X-ray films can have emulsion coated on both sides of film base or only on one side of film base:

- *Double emulsion:* Emulsion is coated on both sides of film base (Fig. 5.1). Now a days double emulsion films are used routinely in X-ray department.
- *Single emulsion:* Emulsion is coated on one side of film. These types of films are used in mammography

In single coated films there is a notch on the film. The emulsion side is facing towards the observer when the notch is in upper right hand corner.

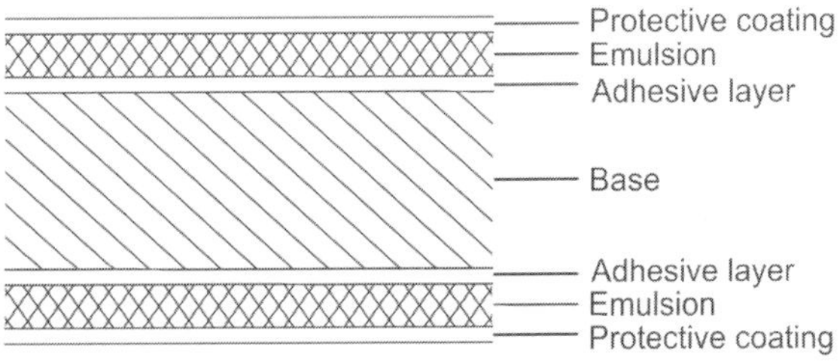

Fig. 5.1 Double emulsion film advantage of film screen over plain X-ray film

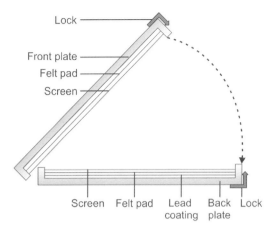

Fig. 5.2 Structure of a cassette

CASSETTE

A cassette is a flat, light proof container for X-ray films, containing front and back intensifying screens, between which the film is placed; for exposure to ionizing radiation and usually backed by lead to eliminate the effects of back scatter radiation. Cassettes are used in association with intensifying screens and screen films.

Basic functions of cassette are:
- To hold a film
- To exclude light for light proof environment
- To maintain the film in close, uniform contact with both screens during the exposure
- To protect the intensifying screens from physical damage.

The standard cassette consists of two flat rectangular plates hinged along one edge. The front aspect of the cassette faces the X-ray tube and consists of a sturdy metal frame into which is fixed a sheet of either light metal such as aluminum, or plastic material which allows transport of X-ray beam. The back of the cassette is constructed from a strong metal. It is customary to spray the internal surface of the back of the cassette with lead paint to absorb secondary radiation, preventing it from being scattered back onto the film. The front and back of the cassette are held tightly together, either by spring clips on the edge opposite to the hinge or by means of pivoted resilient metal bars on the back of the cassette (Fig. 5.2).

The weight of cassette should be light for easy manipulation. As the cassettes in daily use are subject to considerable stress and wear it should have robust structure.

Treated with care X-ray cassettes and intensifying screens are good for years of hard work. Cassettes should be inspected at regular intervals to maintain them in serviceable condition. Hinges and clips are subject to stress and their proper functioning should be checked frequently to assure that wear has not occurred. Loose screens are an invitation to error in the darkroom. Cassettes must be cleaned from inside to avoid dust particles to cause errors. It should be closed only after drying.

Computed radiography (CR) uses a photostimulable phosphor as the image receptor. A phosphor that is currently used is composed of europium-activated barium fluorohalide. The phosphor crystals are coated on a screen that looks like an intensifying screen. The phosphor coated screen is contained in a cassette similar to standard film-screen cassettes. A radiographic exposure is made using conventional X-ray equipment, but here the similarity to conventional radiography ends. The photostimulable phosphor absorbs some of the energy in the X-ray beam and stores a portion of this energy as valence electrons stored in high energy traps to create a latent image. When this latent image is scanned by a laser beam.

Intensifying Screens Used in Cassettes

Intensifying screens used in cassettes consists of fluorescent material, and is placed in contact with the film in a radiographic cassette. Radiation interacts with the fluorescent phosphor in the screen, releasing light photons. These photons expose the film with greater efficiency than would the radiation alone (Fig. 5.3) Thus patient exposure to radiation can be reduced. Phosphors are materials which convert photon energy to light.

The purpose of intensifying screens is to amplify the film blackening effect on the film of an X-ray exposure by the conversion of X-ray photons to light photons to which the film emulsion is sensitive. This depends on the efficiency of the screen phosphor to absorb X-ray photons and convert them to ultra violet and visible light to which the film emulsion is optimally sensitized.

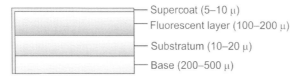

Fig. 5.3 Advantage of film screen over plain X-ray film

The "luminescence" effect is used in screens. It can be described as the emission of light by a substance when excited by any form of energy. When certain materials absorb various kinds of energy, some of the energy may be emitted as light. This process involves two steps:

1. The initial energy causes the electrons of the atoms of the absorbing material to become excited and jump from the inner orbits of the atoms to the outer orbits.
2. When the electrons fall back to their original state, a photon of light is emitted. The interval between the two steps may be short or long. If the interval is short, the process is called fluorescence; if the interval is long, the process is called phosphorescence.

Structure of Intensifying Screen (Fig. 5.4): Intensifying Screen

- *Super coat or the protective layer:* A strong smooth protective layer of cellulose acetate covering and sealing the whole screen, resistant to abrasion, moisture protecting the fluorescent layer, minimal thickness reduces image unsharpness.
- *Fluorescent layer:* An even coating of microscopic phosphor dispersed and suspended in a binding material, e.g. Cellulose acetate. Some phosphor materials are hygroscopic so need to be sealed in; by coating all sides dimensional stability is maintained.
- *Substratum layer:* There are 2 types of substratum both of which may be present and in some case there is no substratum layer and the function is incorporated into the phosphor layer.
  - *Reflective layer:* In order to maximise the amount of light emitted by the phosphor layer a bright white reflective layer is placed between the base and the phosphor layer to reflect as much of the light produced towards the film.
  - *Absorptive layer:* In order to minimise the halation effect (indistinctness of the image caused by illumination coming from the same direction as the object being viewed) hence minimise unsharpness caused by halation. There is sometimes an inert light

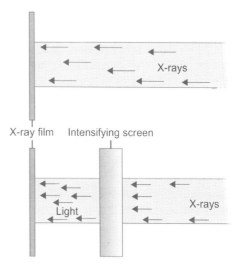

Fig. 5.4 Structure of an intensifying screen

absorptive dye placed between the base and the phosphor to minimise internal reflections within the screen. Absorptive layers which control the screens light output can be used to match screens into a graduated series for specialist applications such as multisection tomography.

- *Base layer:* The base layer acts as a support for the other layers and common materials include card, polyester and plastic. The substratum layer is sometimes incorporated into the base. All layers have to be designed or treated to adhere strongly together.

Phosphors in screens: Standard screens use calcium tungstate phosphors, while rare earth screens use gadolinium or lanthanum phosphors. The commercial name for rare earth screens is Lane. Rare earth phosphors are more efficient at converting X-rays to visible light thus reducing the radiation further to the patient.

Desirable features of phosphors are:

- High X-ray absorption efficiency
- High X-ray to light efficiency
- Emission spectra matched to film sensitivity
- Fast light emission
- Absence of afterglow
- Uniform light output, i.e. uniform dispersion in suspension media.

Types of Phosphors

Early phosphors mainly blue emitters around 380–420 nm. Calcium Tungstate, Silver Zinc Sulphide, Barium lead sulfate, is now superseded in most cases by the "rare earth" phosphors. Lanthanide Series or Rare Earth Elements, series of chemical elements of the periodic table. The rare earth elements (or rare earth metals) include the elements with atomic numbers 57–71. Terbium and Europium are used as activators. Oxysulfides of Gadolinium (Gd), Yttrium (Y) and Lanthanum (La) are most commonly used. The function of the activator is to enhance the light output both in speed and the wavelength of the light to match the application of the screens use.

Speed of Intensifying Screen

There are three types of intensifying screens:
1. *Fast screens:* Rare earth
2. *Slow screens:* Standard
3. *Medium screens:* Combination

- *Fast screens:* They have a thick layer of phosphor and relatively large crystals are used, maximum speed is attained but with some sacrifice in definition.
  Rare earth screen: An intensifying screen is a plastic sheet coated with fluorescent material called phosphors. Phosphors are materials which convert photon energy to light. Rare earth screens are fluorescent screen containing rare earths as the fluorescent material. Crystalline lanthanum and gadolinium are used in several rare earth screens, but rare earth phosphors in general show little fluorescence in the pure state. When some of the rare earth atoms in a pure crystalline rare earth phosphor are replaced by another rare earth element (an impurity or activating substance), a high degree of fluorescence is achieved. As compared to the traditional calcium tungstate intensifying screen, the rare earth screens have about four times as high X-ray to light conversion efficiency, and also a higher X-ray absorption efficiency. Due to the high atomic number of the screen phosphors, X-ray absorption is almost entirely due to photoelectric absorption. Photoelectric absorption in an atom decreases steadily with increasing X-ray energy, but increases abruptly at the K edge of the atom. Lanthanum and gadolinium have K edges at 38. 9 and 50. 2 keV, respectively. Most X-ray spectra used in conventional skeletal imaging have a mean energy between 40 and 50 keV, making especially lanthanum much more effective in absorbing these energies than tungsten (some gadolinium screens have added lanthanum for this reason). On the other hand, due to the effective photoelectric absorption at these energies, somewhat more characteristic radiation is liberated in the rare earth screens as compared to calcium tungstate screens. This tends to decrease the contrast information available with the rare earth screens. Rare earth screens emit light in narrow lines with very strong peak(s) in the green part of the spectrum, but also smaller ones in the blue, blue-green and yellow areas. The term "green screen" is used. They require special green sensitive film and special darkroom safe light.

- *Slow screens or high definition screens:* They have a thin layer of phosphor and relatively small crystals are used; shows good details, but speed is slow necessitating a higher dose of ionizing radiation.

- *Medium screens:* They have a medium thick layer of medium sized phosphor crystals in order to provide comprise between speed and definition.

  Screen speed is a separate measured quantity to film speed or film screen combination speed. Generally this is expressed in terms of the amount luminance for a given X-ray exposure. There is increasing support for a relative speed indication system where a reference screen is set at 100 and others have their speed indicted relative to this, i.e. 200 requiring half the X-ray exposure to produce the same level of luminance. The methods which increase screen cause a change in other factors such as image sharpness and contrast. It must be remembered that any indication of comparative screen speed must be for identical exposure conditions especially the kV and the voltage waveforms of the generator.

  Screen speed may be increased by the following methods.

- Selection of an efficient phosphor/activator combination.
- Increasing phosphor particle size (up to point)
- Minimizing the binder volume
- Increasing the phosphor layer thickness
- Employing a reflective layer.

Functioning of Intensifying Screen

Each crystal on the screen emits bluish light for regular screens (or green light for rare earth screens). Brightness is related directly to the intensity of the X-rays in that minute portion of the image. Thus, over the entire surface of the screen, differences in X-ray intensities are transformed into differences of bluish light (green light) brightness to which the film is highly sensitive. The entire image is thus intensified for recording by the film. The larger the crystals and the thicker the fluorescent layer on the screen, the more light is produced and the greater the intensification. However, the light spreads more widely and the sharpness of detail of the image is decreased accordingly.

Image Contrast

Screen influence on image contrast is one of the principal influences on image contrast the others include exposure Kv and generator waveform and film properties patient type.

Screen contrast is affected by

- X-ray photon kV.
- Phosphor type
- Speed difference between front and back screen.

Image Sharpness

Radiographic unsharpness is determined by the three factors.

1. Movement unsharpness
2. Geometric unsharpness
3. Film screen combination unsharpness, including the related film screen contact element.

The following five methods increase screen sharpness but must be considered with the other influences.

1. Decreasing phosphor layer thickness
2. Decreasing phosphor particle size
3. Maximizing protective layer transparency
4. Addition of absorptive dyes to the phosphor layer
5. Omitting the reflective layer.

Care of Screens

Screens should be cleaned as per the manufactures recommendations with particular regard to the use of solvent cleaners which may damage the protective coating.

In general any dust and particles should be blown out, the cassette should then be brushed out with a soft paintbrush then a lightly moistened cotton wool ball should be wiped gently across the surface, then the same with a dry one. Finally the cassette should be left open on its edge to dry in a convenient place.

- Do not scratch at any surface.
- Do not make the screen wet.
- Do not use unproved solvents.
- Ensure the screen is fully dry before reloading the cassette.
- Record the date of cleaning.

Increasing Film Speed

- Thicker phosphor layers.
- Higher conversion efficiency.
- Higher absorption phosphor.
- Decreased resolution of image.

PROCESSING OF EXPOSED X-RAY FILMS

After the films are exposed to radiation, they need to be processed in order to see the information on the film to convert latent image to manifest image. For this the films need to be processed. There are two types of processing

1. Wet processing
2. Dry processing

Wet processing can be manual or automatic.

Advantages of dry over wet processing are that it provides less plumbing costs, no chemicals and hence less environmental pollution and reduced maintenance.

Advantages of automatic over manual processing are that manual processing is very time and labor intensive, requiring a much longer processing time than automatic processing and requiring someone to be available to transfer films into the various solutions. Drying films also takes time.

Wet Processing

Manual Processing

With manual processing, two tanks, one containing developer and one fixer, are placed in a larger tank filled with water. The water is maintained at a certain temperature using a mixing valve. The film is first placed in the developer for a specified time, rinsed in the water, and then placed in the fixer. After fixing for the appropriate time, the film is washed in the water. The overflow tube prevents water from rising high enough to enter the developer or fixer tanks. For manual processing, films are clipped to some type of film hanger. The film should be handled only by the edges to avoid damage. The film hanger, with films attached, is then placed in the processing solutions, developer first. The approximate time films are kept in different solutions is as follows:

Develop: 5 minutes at 68 degrees (agitate gently)

Rinse: 30 seconds (agitate continuously)

Fix: 4 minutes (agitate intermittently)

Wash: 10 minutes in clean running water

After completion of manual processing films are hanged on hangers to dry.

Developing of X-ray Films (Table 5.1)

The components of compound of developer and their functions are as follows.

Two important factors in development are the temperature of developing solution and total time of development. Optimum temperature of developing solution should be maintained between 60°F and 70°F. If the solution is colder of hotter it results in chemical fogging.

Replenishment: It important to replenish the strength and volume of developing solution. Developing

Table 5.1 Components of developer and their functions

Component	Chemical	Function
Developing agent	Phenindone Hydroquinone	Produce shades of black and gray
Preservative	Sodium sulfite	Protects reducing agent from oxidation by air
Restrained	Potassium bromide	Prevents action of developing agent on unexposed crystal
Accelerator	Sodium hydroxide or Sodium carbonate	Controls pH (alkaline) helps swell gelatine
Solvent	Water	Dissolve chemical for use

Table 5.2 Components of fixer and their functions

Component	Chemical	Function
Fixing agent	Sodium thiosulfate (powder) Ammonium Thiosulfate	Remove undeveloped and unexposed silver bromide
Hardener	Potassium hydroxide	Stiffen and shrink solution
Preservative	Sodium sulfite	Protects reducing agent from oxidation by air
Accelerator	Sulfuric acid	Neutralizes alkali from film and maintains pH
Solvent	Water	Dissolve other components

solution diminishes as reducing agents are gradually exhausted in the process of development. The constituents of replenisher are
- Hydroquinone, metol and alkali as these are exhausted during process of development.
- No bromide as this accumulates in developing solution during process of development.

Rinsing

After development film is suspended in rinsing bath for 30 seconds. Rinsing is required for removing traces of developer from film as the presence of developer would quickly deprive fixer of its effectiveness and give rise to film fog. Without rinsing the fixer does not act evenly and gives rise to film fog. Rinsing is omitted in automatic processing.

Fixing (Table 5.2)

The purpose of fixation is to remove undeveloped and unexposed silver halide, to harden the emulsion so

that it is not easily damaged and to preserve the film image. The components of fixing solution and their functions are as follows.

Rapid fixer is used to reduce the fixing time, it contains ammonium chloride and is used in automatic processors.

Washing

It is done to wash away any residual fixing agent to the solution as residual fixing agent can change black silver to brown silver sulfide. Washing requires running water at approximately 20°C.

Drying

It is the final step in processing. The films must be hanged in dust free area and the temperature must not exceed 35°C.

Automatic Processing

The basic mechanism of this type of processing is a series of rollers which transport films through various sections. The speed of rollers and their spacing must be accurate to ensure optimum performance. Chemicals of automatic processor differ from those of manual processor in certain aspects. Increased concentration of phenindone and hydroquinone to decrease processing time.

Increase in hardness of emulsion by adding potassium bromide to prevent softening and sticking of films by rollers.

Increase in temperatures of processing unit to speed up the process. Antifogging agents (aldehyde) are added to developer to prevent film fogging. Controlling emulsion thickness to keep it constant throughout the process. Sulfates are added to developer for this to reduce the swelling of emulsion. Precise replenishment of developer to maintain alkalinity of developer and acidity of fixer. In automatic processors agitation of films is provided by circulating system which pumps the developer and fixer. Fresh water is piped into the tank at bottom and it overflows out at the top where it is directly taken into sewer system.

The rollers must be thoroughly clean and automatic replenishes must be precise to maintain processor functioning.

Processing Errors (Darkroom Film Artifacts)

- *Film density:* The density of the film can be affected by problems in the darkroom, resulting in a film that is too light or too dark. A dark film can result from any of the following:

If
- Developer too hot
- Too much time in the developer
- Exposure to light (opening door, turning on light, light leaks around door, incorrect or cracked filters).

If the films are kept in the developer for the correct amount of time but the developer is too hot, the film will get darker as the temperature increases. If the films are kept in the developer too long, even though the temperature is correct, the film will get darker as the time increases. Opening the door during processing could also create a dark film. Light leaks or faulty safe lighting would result in an overall darkening of the film, similar to too high a temperature.

- A light film can result from any of the following:
  - Developer too cold
  - Not enough time in the developer
  - Under replenishment (developer gets weak)
  - Contaminated developer
  - Excessive fixation

- *Dark spots due to developer contamination:* If drops of developer accidentally contact the film prior to processing, the developing action will start to act on these areas immediately. When the film is then placed in the developer, the overall time that these areas are developed is longer than for the rest of the film, resulting in darker spots.

- *Light spots due to fixer contamination:* If drops of fixer accidentally contact the film prior to processing, the fixing action will start to act on these areas immediately. When the film is then placed in the developer, there are fewer crystals to be converted to black metallic silver, resulting in lighter spots. Usually the contamination is on one side of the film only so that the crystals in the emulsion on the opposite side are processed normally and you can still see part of the image.

- *Yellow or brown stain due to depleted fixer:* If the film is not adequately fixed, the undeveloped crystals (those without exposure centers) will not be removed from the film, resulting in a yellowish-brown stain. This is more apparent in the film below in the areas that were not exposed to X-rays.

- *Films overlapped during processing:* If films are fed into the automatic processor too quickly, the films may overlap each other, preventing the processing chemicals from acting on the overlapped emulsions. This results in a dark area on each film.

- *Film fogging:* If there is light leak or improper safe lighting in the darkroom, the film may be fogged before being processed. Film fogging is the exposure of more of the silver halide crystals than would normally be affected during the taking of a radiograph. The exposure of these extra crystals results in the film being darker than normal and will usually decrease the diagnostic value of the film. If a film is processed without being exposed to light or X-rays, it should come out completely clear (white on the view box). A fogged film will have an overall slight greyness.

Automatic Film Processor Artifacts

- Water spots can occur on the film if the replenishment rates are incorrect, if the squeeze mechanism that the film passes through after the wash tank is defective, or if the dryer is malfunctioning. Water spots are best seen with reflected light.

- A slap line is a plus-density line perpendicular to the direction of film travel that occurs near the trailing edge of the film. This is caused by the abrupt release of the back edge of the film as it passes through the developer-to-fixer crossover assembly.

- Pick-off artifacts are small, clear areas of the film where emulsion has flecked off from the film base; they can be caused by rough rollers, no uniform film transport, or a mismatch between the film emulsion and chemicals.

- Wet pressure marks occur when the pinch rollers apply too much or inconsistent pressure to the film in the developer or in the developer-to-fixer crossover racks.

- Shoe marks result when the film rubs against the guide shoes during transport. The artifact manifests as a series of evenly spaced lines parallel the direction of film transport.

- *Run back artifacts:* Fluid drops at trailing edge of the film.

- *Chatter:* Set of lines occurring periodically perpendicular to film transport direction caused by binding of roller assembly in developer fixer crossover assembly or a developer tank.

Dry Processing

Dry processors, like laser cameras, are used for producing images from digital modalities, such as X-ray ultrasound, digital radiography, CT, and MR. The imaging plate is exposed in a procedure identical to screen film radiography, and the CR cassette is then brought to a CR reader unit. The cassette is placed in the readout unit, and several processing steps then take place:

- The cassette is moved into the reader unit and the imaging plate is mechanically removed from the cassette.
- The imaging plate is translated across a moving stage and scanned by a laser beam.
- The laser light stimulates the emission of trapped energy in the imaging plate, and visible light is released from the plate.
- The light released from the plate is collected by a fibre optic light guide and strikes a photomultiplier tube (PMT), where it produces an electronic signal.
- The electronic signal is digitized and stored.
- The plate is then exposed to bright white light to erase any residual trapped energy.
- The imaging plate is then returned to the cassette and is ready for reuse.

Quality Control (Factors Affecting Quality of Radiograph)

X-ray film: The film should to be used before its expiry date and stored appropriately.

Processing: Optimal performance needs to be evaluated daily using quality control tests.

X-ray units: These need to be inspected by a qualified expert at regular intervals to ensure proper performance.

Technique: The operator must use proper technique in taking films.

Benefits of Quality Control

- *Improved diagnosis:* If the quality of the films is optimized, the films will provide the best diagnostic information.
- *Reduced patient exposure:* If the X-ray machine is working properly and no retakes are needed (due to faulty technique or processing), patient exposure will be minimized.
- *Time and cost savings:* If everything is done properly, and no retakes are necessary, the operator won't need to devote excess time to retaking films and fewer films will be used.

Quality Control Tests

Quality control tests are primarily used to identify problems with the processing of films but may also identify problems with the X-ray equipment. Quality control tests include:
- *Reference radiograph:* A properly exposed and processed film is kept on the view box. Each day a new film is exposed and processed and compared to the reference radiograph. Differences in the films may indicate a problem.
  This is the least reliable test.
- *Step wedge:* An aluminum step wedge with varying thicknesses of aluminum (steps) is placed on a film packet and exposed with standard exposure settings. It is then processed under ideal conditions (processor cleaned with new solutions). Each day a new film is exposed and processed using the step wedge. These daily films are compared to the original (ideal) film. If the steps on the daily film line up with the steps on the original film (same densities) the test is considered negative. This indicates that everything is satisfactory and no changes are needed.

If the steps on the daily film do not line up with the steps on the original film (different densities) the test is considered positive. This indicates that there is a problem that needs to be corrected. The most likely problem is with processing. If you clean the processor and add new solutions and the steps on a new film still do not line up, the problem is probably with the X-ray equipment.

DRY IMAGING CAMERAS

Dry imaging cameras are also known as dry imaging devices, laser printers, direct digital imagers or hard copy cameras. Dry imaging cameras are widely used in laser optic technologies. In dry view camera the development process is accomplished by heating a dry film a process known as photothermography.

It is a two-step process. It involves a laser diode optic system and photothermography. The latent image which is created by using either optics or heat is converted into true image by photothermography. The latent image is created by a laser which induces photons in the light sensitive layer of the film which converts silver ions to silver atoms. The latent image depends upon intensity of the laser beam. The film is then transported to a rotating drum where it absorbs energy for 15 sec at a temperature of 120 to 140°C. By a catalytic process thermal energy acts on latent image to develop silver atoms (true image).

Printing in Dry Laser Camera

A suction cup lifts a single film out of supply cartridge and feeds it into vertical transport rollers. The film moves to a film platen which holds the film while the scanner writes the image onto the film. Film transport rollers then move the film to a sorter and then to the bins or at the top of hood.

6

Fluoroscopic Imaging

Prashant Naik

X-rays have ability to cause fluorescence. The basic components of fluoroscope are X-ray tube, X-ray table and fluoroscopic screen.

Fluoroscopic screen contains fluoroscent material. Early fluoroscopes contained copper activated zinc cadmium sulfide as fluoroscopic material in the screen which emitted light when struck by X-rays. An image of the part screened with X-rays is formed on this fluoroscopic screen. This screen is covered with a sheet of lead glass to protect the radiologist standing in front of this screen. However the fluoroscopic image formed is so faint that it can be seen only in dark, that too after dark adaptation by the radiologist by wearing red goggles. This image is perceived by rods (peripheral vision) in human retina. This vision in human eye has poor visual acuity. The image was not bright enough for cones in fovea of the retina to see it clearly. Hence the need for making this image bright enough by some mechanism was felt and finally in the early 1958 the image intensifier was developed.

An X-ray image intensifier is a image vacuum tube which is a highly evacuated glass envelope (2–4 mm thick) enclosed in a metal container lined with lead. It converts a low intensity X-ray image into a visible image. The X-ray image intensifier is generally a cylindrically-shaped device containing a number of components housed in a vacuum.

Image intensifier (Fig. 6.1) has following components
- The *input window* in older intensifiers was made from glass and their performance suffered from X-ray scattering and absorption effects in this material. In modern devices a relatively thin sheet of aluminum or titanium are used with minimal X-ray attenuation.
- *Input phosphor:* X-ray tube emits X-rays that pass through patient and then fall on input phosphor of image intensifier. This input fluorescent screen is made up of cesium fluoride generally cesium iodide (CsI) deposited on aluminum substrate. The early image intensifiers used silver activated zinc-cadmium sulfide. However, the image quality with CsI screens is far superior to older zinc cadmium

sulfide screens due to vertical orientation of crystals, a greater packing density and a more favorable effective atomic number.

Phosphor thickness of CsI is 0.1 mm which is one third of zinc cadmium sulfide. Due to this thinner layer and needle shaped crystals, the resolution substantially improves. CsI input screen absorbs two thirds of incident X-ray beams whereas zinc cadmium sulfide absorbs only one third.
- *Photocathode:* The photocathode is a photo-emissive metal commonly a combination of antimony and cesium compound. It is applied directly to the CsI input phosphor. When photocathode is struck by light from fluorescent screen it emits photoelectrons in numbers proportional to the brightness of the screen. This forms an electronic image duplicated on the light image. The curved design of photocathode enhances sharpness of electronic image. These electrons travel to the output screen of the image

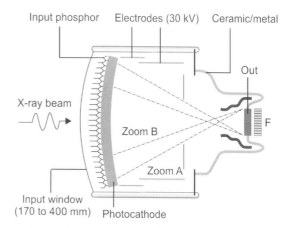

Fig. 6.1 Design of image intensifier in cross-section. X-rays emerging from the patient enter at the input window and strike the input phosphor. The input phosphor scintillates and light photons produced strike the photocathode, which emits electrons. These electrons are accelerated and focused by the electron optics onto the output phosphor which emits light. This light provides an image of the X-ray pattern that emerged from the patient which has a substantially greater intensity than when an intensifying screen if used on its own

intensifier tube. However to maintain their relative position in the beam; this beam has to be focused by electrostatic focusing lens and accelerating anode.

- *Electrostatic focusing lens* is nothing but positively charged electrodes coated on inside of the glass tube which focus the electron beam towards the output phosphor. Due to focusing the image on output phosphor is reduced in size and hence it becomes brighter.

  Vacuum is required so that the electrons can travel unimpeded—as in the case of the X-ray tube. A voltage of 25 to 35 kV is used to accelerate the electrons and the electron optics is used for focusing them onto the output phosphor. A current of about 10^{-8} to 10^{-7} A results and it is the acceleration and focusing of these electrons which gives rise to the image intensification.

  Accelerating anode is placed in the neck of the tube that accelerates the electrons from photocathode to output screen.

- *Output phosphor* is made of silver activated zinc-cadmium sulfide. Size of the output screen is about 2.5 cm. The number of light photons emitted here are about 50 times more than the input screen as the electrons are highly accelerated. A thin aluminum layer on this fluorescent screen prevents light from moving backwards into the tube. And thus the image is finally displayed on output screen.

This output screen of the image intensifier can be seen directly by the view through a series of lenses and mirrors or through closed circuit television indirectly. Closed circuit television is used in most of the modern image intensifiers (I.I.). Thus the fluorescent image resulting on output phosphor is much brighter than input image, i.e. brightness gain due to following reasons.

- Electron acceleration (Fluoro gain)
- Small size of output phosphor in comparison with input phosphor (Minification gain).

Brightness is increased at the output phosphor 50 times to that of input phosphor due to electron acceleration so the flux is gain is about 50.

Minification gain $(dI/do)\,2$. Where dI is diameter of input screen and do is diameter of output screen

Brightness gain = minification gain × flux gain

This images recorded are continuously viewed on output phosphor image on TV; the light from image intensifier output screen can be split into two directions by a semitransparent mirror which is placed in the path of light beam. Part of light goes to TV and part goes to film camera. So that recording and viewing of the image can go on simultaneously.

FACTORS AFFECTING IMAGE QUALITY

Two factor that reduce contrast in image intensifier are:

- The input screen does not absorb all the photons in the X-ray beam. Some are transmitted through the intensifier tube and they along with electrons emitted from input phosphor.

  A few of then ultimately reach the output screen. They along with electrons emitted from input phosphor also illuminate output phosphor, but do not contribute to image formation. They produce background fog which reduces image contrast.

After the electrons strike output phosphor, there is some retrograde light flow from it which passes back through the image tube and activates photocathode. In turn it emits photoelectrons which come back to output phosphor and produces fog. Most of this retrograde flow is prevented by a thin aluminum layer. Some light photons still penetrate to produce fog by a process explained earlier.

LAG

X-rays stimulate the phosphor and cause luminescence which is seen as image. However luminescence of phosphor screen continues for some time even after the X-ray stimulation is terminated. This is called lag. Lag time is about 1 ms in CsI screen.

DISTORTION

As the electron beam is emitted from photocathode and travel toward the output screen, electric fields controlling the direction and speed of electrons can accurately control the electrons in the center of the beam, however peripheral electrons cannot be controlled so accurately and they deviate from their path and are not properly focused on the output phosphor. Hence there is some amount of distortion in the periphery of the image. This effect is called pincushion effect. Unequal magnification leads to unequal illumination of output screen. This results in the image being brighter at center and dimmer at periphery. This phenomenon is called vignetting.

These effects are more pronounced in larger field image intensifier.

MULTIPLE FIELD IMAGE INTENSIFIERS

These image intensifiers (Fig. 6.1) can be used in different modes, e.g. 4.5″, 6″, or 9″, larger field, i.e. 12″ to 16″ are also available. Smaller the size, better is the image quality.

CINEFLUOROGRAPHY

Fluoroscopic imaging procedure can be recorded in real time on cine film. A series of lenses and mirrors are placed between the output phosphor of the image intensifier and cine camera. The image is thus relayed to the camera which records it. Simultaneous television viewing and recording is achieved by a beam-splitting mirror.

Cinefluorography is very valuable for recording the movement of a contrast agent through vessels. A lens, iris-diaphragm, shutter, aperture, pressure plate, pull down arm, film transport mechanism are the basic components of conventional camera.

Lens of the camera allows light to enter it, which is controlled by the aperture over it. Aperture is an opening in the front of the camera. Aperture size and shape can be changed manually or electronically which defines the configuration of the image that reaches the film. A film reel having two parts (a supply reel and take up reel) is mounted behind the aperture. An electronic drive motor rotates the reel and the film behind the aperture advances from the supply reel to take up reel and the real time images from output phosphor are recorded on this moving film. Typically it is recorded at 15, 30, 60 and 90 frames per second.

In all modern cinefluorographic systems open time of camera shutter is synchronized with the intermittent X-ray output on the phosphor.

Modern video recorders are now used in place of conventional film cameras for recording the fluorography procedures. Digital imaging sensor is used here in place of conventional photographic film. And the digitized video images thus grabbed can be stored on Digital Versatile Disc or Digital Video Disc (DVD). These digital video clips can be stored in computer hard disc or other types of modern data storage devices also for future reference.

7

Image Quality

Roshan Lodha

Radiographic image quality refers to the visible sharpness of images of structural details. Recorded detail refers to the distinctness of radiographic image margins. When margins are blurred, recorded detail is poor. Sharpness of image margins is noted by the abruptness of the boundary between a detail and its surrounding. The principal factors that influence recorded detail are blur, density, contrast and distortion .

BLUR

There are four causes of image blurring or unsharpness:
1. Geometric or focal spot blur
2. Motion blur
3. Screen blur
4. Object blur.

- *Geometric or focal spot blur:* The term penumbra can be used as synonym for geometric blur.

    Penumbra is lack of sharpness (unsharpness) of the film often termed as edge gradient. It is the region of partial illumination that surrounds the umbra or complete shadow. It is a fuzzy, unclear area that surrounds a radiographic image. Focal spot has finite dimension and each point on focal spot acts as if it were composed of many point sources of X-rays, with each point source forming its own image of an object. The edges of each image formed will not be in exactly same spot on film and thus producing image unsharpness.

    Penumbra depends on three factors: Effective focal spot size, focus film distance, and object film distance. Tubes with smaller focal spot provide better recorded detail, with resulting improved image quality. Recorded detail, i.e. image sharpness is enhanced by any factor that decreases geometric blur or penumbra, namely, small tube focus, long focus film distance and short object film distance. Part to be radiographed should be placed as close to the film as possible and appropriate long focus film distance with smallest focal spot should be used.

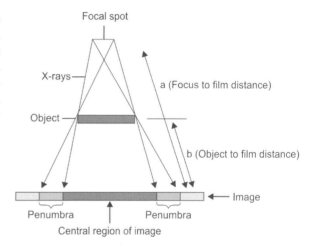

Fig. 7.1 Geometric or focal spot blur or penumbra

Geometric or focal spot blur or penumbra is reduced by small tube focus, long focus-film distance and short object – film distance (Fig. 7.1). Penumbra is calculated by

$$Ug = f \times b/a$$

f = X-ray generator focal-spot size.

a = distance from X-ray source to front surface of material/object

b = distance from the material/object to the detector.

- *Motion blur:* Motion of the part being radio-graphed produces a blurred image. Motion can be minimized by careful immobilization of the part with sand bags or compression band, by suspension of respiration when examining parts other than the limbs and by using exposures that are as short as possible, generally with intensifying screens of adequate speed.

- *Screen blur:* Screen blur is generally of the order of about six times inherent film blur. Blur with medium speed screens is about one half that with high speed screens. Blur with high and medium speed films is virtually negligible in radiography. Screen blur increases with increasing crystal size and with increasing thickness of active layer of fluorescent crystals. Even a slight separation between film and screen contributes to blur with impaired recorded detail. Slow screen film systems should be used in the radiography of small parts, especially in infants and small children. In the radiography of parts measuring 8 to 10 cm thick, medium or high speed screen should be used routinely; and above 10 cm, a grid also. Radiograph exposed by means of screen show a mottled or grainy appearance. Quantum mottle is produced by the nonuniform intensity over the cross section of an X-ray beam as it leaves the tube port. Quantum mottle increases with high contrast films because density differences are exaggerated. High kV increases quantum mottle.

- *Object blur:* If shape of the object conforms to that of the beam, the density trace is sharp at the edges. Progressively smaller thickness of the object intercepts the beam toward the edge, so the density falls off gradually at the image boundary, which is therefore less sharp than objects which conforms the shape of the beam.

DENSITY

The amount of darkening of an X-ray film, or a certain area on the film, is called radiographic density. The radiographic density depends on the amount of radiation reaching a particular area of the film and the resulting mass of metallic silver deposited per unit area during development. Density is an extremely important factor in radiographic quality because it carries information. Without density there is no image and therefore no recorded detail. Five factors govern the radiation exposure and resulting density of a radiograph: kilovoltage, milliamperage, time, distance, thickness and nature of part being examined. An increase in kV increases the exposure rate at the film and resulting radiographic density. Doubling the mA doubles the radiographic exposure rate. Doubling the time doubles the total exposure. Radiographic exposure rate decreases as the focus film distance increases. Thicker and denser anatomic part, whether normal or pathological, attenuate X-rays to greater degree, leaving less remnant radiation to reach the film.

CONTRAST

The range of density variation among the light and dark areas is called radiographic contrast. Radiographic contrast depends on subject contrast and film contrast. Subject contrast depends on thickness difference, density difference, atomic number difference, and radiation quality (kVp). Increase in kV produces lower contrast resulting from the increase in the fraction of scattered radiation. Greater the attenuation coefficient of a given type of tissues, less its radiolucency and the smaller the amount of transmitted or exit radiation reaching the film. Scatter radiation impairs contrast by a fogging effect mainly on light areas of the radiograph. Fogging from any cause contributes to noise, imparting an overall gray appearance to the radiograph with reduction in contrast. Film contrast depends on type of image receptor, its use with or without screens, and the processing system. Films themselves vary in their inherent contrast, depending on their emulsion characteristics. Development process also affects the film contrast.

DISTORTION

Misinterpretation of the true size and shape of an object is called distortion. There are two kinds of distortion—size distortion and shape distortion. Size distortion or magnification is due to the divergence of the X-rays in the beam. The law of image magnification states that the width of the image is to the width of the object as the distance of the image from the light source is to the distance of the object from the light source. Six feet focus film distance is used to minimize the cardiac magnification. Magnification or size distortion can be minimized either by reducing the object film distance or by increasing the focus film distance. Shape distortion result from improper alignment of the central ray, object, and film.

8

Radiation Hazards and Protection

Amol Sasane

In the environment there is continuous radiation, which is both natural and artificial. The natural sources include cosmic radiation from space, radiation from the earth and its internal radionuclide. Artificial sources of radiation include X-ray equipment, nuclear weapons and radioactive medication.

Radiation is energy in transit in the form of high speed particles and electromagnetic waves. Radiation can be ionizing or nonionizing. X-rays are electromagnetic waves or photons not emitted from the nucleus, but normally emitted by energy changes in electrons. These energy changes are either in electron orbital shells that surround an atom or in the process of slowing down such as in an X-ray machine.

Roentgen discovered X-rays in November 1895, after that X-rays are used globally. Initial hazards of radiation reported were eye complaints and severe progressive dermatitis. Clarence E Dally developed ulcerating carcinoma of his left hand in 1896. He was involved in the production of X-ray tubes, where he was using his own hand to test their output. Delayed effects of radiation began to be documented only 20 years after their initial discovery, through individual case reports.

CLASSIFICATION OF RADIATION INJURY

Radiation effects are classified as: Directly proportional to dose, i.e. deterministic effects, or not directly proportional to dose, i.e. stochastic effects.

- *Somatic*
  - *Deterministic effects:* Deterministic effects are related with certainty to a known dose of radiation. There is threshold to the dose of radiation. In these the severity is dose related and includes cataracts, blood dyscrasias and impaired fertility.
  - *Stochastic effects:* Stochastic effects are random effects without threshold. In these probability increases with dose, and severity may not be dose related and includes cancer and genetic effects.
- *Genetic:* These are always stochastic effects.

Deterministic Health Effects

Exposure to high levels of radiation leads to deterministic (nonstochastic) health effects. These effects depend on the dose of the radiation the person is exposed to. Greater the exposure, more severe is the damage. Short-term, high-level exposure is referred to as "acute" exposure. Health effects produced by an 'acute' exposure to radiation occur quickly. Nonstochastic health effects are mostly noncancerous. The most important health effects are burns and radiation sickness. Radiation Sickness (radiation poisoning) can cause premature aging or even death. Exposure to fatal doses can lead to death.

Some symptoms of radiation sickness are nausea, weakness, hair loss, skin burns, diminished organ function.

Relatively high "bursts" of radiation that patients receive during medical treatment often cause acute effects. Neutropenia due to radiation exposure can occur.

Somatic certainty effects which have been evaluated on patients undergoing radiotherapy have shown that the tissues most sensitive to radiation damage are bone marrow, eye and gonads. From studies on radiotherapy patients, the threshold doses are estimated at 1 Gy (Gray) for bone marrow, 2–8 Gy for eye, 3–4 Gy to elicit ovulation failure in middle aged women and 6-10 Gy cause failure of spermatogenesis. It has been found that the GIT is sensitive at 75 Gy, the brain beyond 55-60 Gy, the spinal cord at 45 Gy, the heart at 40-50 Gy and the lung at 11 Gy.

Stochastic Effects

Cancer is the uncontrolled growth of cells. Cell division is a fundamental process that takes place in the human body. A multitude of mechanisms exist to ensure that this process occur error free and in strict control. Damage occurring at the cellular or molecular level can disrupt this and lead to uncontrolled proliferation of cells. Ionizing radiation has the ability to break chemical bonds in atoms and molecules. Owing to this potential, it may be referred to as a carcinogen. Cancer is commonly considered as the primary health effect from radiation exposure.

Malignancies because of radiation exposure are leukemias, carcinoma of lung, breast, thyroid and skin and meningiomas and osteosarcomas. Effects on the fetus are both deterministic and stochastic which lead to childhood malignancies. Irradiation *in utero* can lead to developmental abnormalities (more during 8–25 weeks of gestation), and cancer may develop during childhood or as adult.

However since radiation exposure has inherent risks of radiation effects, no decision to expose an individual can be undertaken without weighing benefits of exposure against potential risks. That is, making a benefit risk analysis.

Radiation Units

Roentgen is a unit used to measure a quantity called exposure. One roentgen is equal to depositing in dry air enough energy to cause 2.58×10^{-4} coulombs per kg. It is a measure of the ionizations of the molecules in a mass of air.

Rad (radiation absorbed dose) is a unit used to measure a quantity called absorbed dose. This relates to the amount of energy actually absorbed in some material, and is used for any type of radiation and any material. One rad is defined as the absorption of 100 ergs per gram of material.

Rem (roentgen equivalent man) is a unit used to derive a quantity called equivalent dose. This relates the absorbed dose in human tissue to the effective biological damage of the radiation. Equivalent dose is often expressed in terms of thousandths of a rem, or mrem. To determine equivalent dose (rem), you multiply absorbed dose (rad) by a quality factor (Q) that is unique to the type of incident radiation.

Curie (Ci) is a unit used to measure a radioactivity. One curie is that quantity of a radioactive material that will have 37,000,000,000 transformations in one second. The relationship between Becquerel and curies is: 3.7×10^{10} Bq in one curie.

Gray (Gy) is a unit used to measure a quantity called absorbed dose. This relates to the amount of energy actually absorbed in some material, and is used for any type of radiation and any material. One gray is equal to one joule of energy deposited in one kg of a material. Absorbed dose is often expressed in terms of hundredths of a gray, or centi-grays. One gray is equivalent to 100 rads.

Becquerel (Bq) is a unit used to measure a radioactivity. One Becquerel is that quantity of a radioactive material that will have 1 transformation in

one second. Often radioactivity is expressed in larger units like: thousands (k Bq), one millions (m Bq) or even billions (g Bq) of a Becquerel. As a result of having one Becquerel being equal to one transformation per second, there are 3.7×10^{10} Bq in one curie.

Sievert (Sv) is a unit used to derive a quantity called equivalent dose. This relates the absorbed dose in human tissue to the effective biological damage of the radiation. Equivalent dose is often expressed in terms of millionths of a sievert, or micro-sievert. To determine equivalent dose (Sv), you multiply absorbed dose (Gy) by a quality factor (Q) that is unique to the type of incident radiation. One sievert is equivalent to 100 rem.

A given material has an ability to absorb radiation when exposed. This differs with certain materials, some will absorb more, e.g. lead or less, e.g. water, as radiation passes through.

Conventional units: A dose of 1 rad means the absorption of 100 ergs of radiation energy per gram of absorbing material.

SI units (abbreviated SI from French: *Système international d'unités*): A dose of 1 gray means the absorption of 1 joule of radiation energy per kilogram of absorbing material.

1 Gy = 100 rads

The dose equivalent is a measure of biological effect for whole body irradiation. It is measured in Sievert (Sv). The dose equivalent is equal to the product of the absorbed dose and the Quality factor (Q).

The Quality Factor depends on the type of radiation. X-ray and Gamma ray the Quality Factor (Q) is 1.

1 Sievert (Sv) = 100 rads. 1 mSv = 0.1 rad

A **röntgen (R)** is an obsolete unit of radiation exposure, which is the measure of the amount of radiation required to create 1 electrostatic unit (esu) of charge of each polarity in 1 cubic centimeter of dry air. 1 röntgen = 0.000258 coulomb/kilogram (C/kg) i.e. 2.58×10^{-4} C/kg.

Radiation levels are measured mSv and other international variants as follows:

- 1 Sv = 1000 mSv = 1,000,000 µSv (microsieverts) = 100 rem = 100,000 mrem (millirem)
- 1 mSv = 100 mrem = 0.1 rem
- 1 µSv = 0.1 mrem
- 1 rem = 0.01 Sv = 10 mSv
- 1 mrem = 0.00001 Sv = 0.01 mSv = 10 µSv
- *1 Roentgen = 1 RAD = 1 REM* 1 rem = 0.01 Sv = 10 mSv = 10 mGy = 0.01 Gy.

During a nuclear disaster the serious *accumulative* radiation danger level is 1 Sv (1000 mSv). This level results in illness and serious health issues or latent death. 100 mSv/hour for 10 hours will gives a total 1000 mSv—the maximum risk level.

The Deciding Authority

The International Commission of Radiation Protection (ICRP) formed in 1928. The ICRP is the international regulatory body. Atomic Energy Regulatory Board (AERB) which is the Indian regulatory board constituted on November 15, 1983. The mission of the Board is to ensure that the use of ionizing radiation and nuclear energy in India does not cause undue risk to health and environment.

AERB recommends and lays down guidelines regarding the specifications of medical X-ray equipment, for the room layout of X-ray installation, regarding the work practices in X-ray department, the protective devices and also the responsibilities of the radiation personnel, employer and Radiation Safety Officer (RSO). It is the authority in India which exercises a regulatory control and has the power to decommissioning X-ray installations and also for imposing penalties on any person contravening these rules.

The Objective of Radiation Protection

Provide an appropriate standard of protection for man without unduly limiting the beneficial practices giving rise to radiation exposure. Current standards of protection are meant to prevent occurrence of deterministic effects by keeping doses below relevant thresholds and ensure that all reasonable steps are taken to reduce induction of stochastic effects.

Optimization of Protection and the ALARA Principle

Optimization of protection can be achieved by optimizing the procedure to administer a radiation dose which is as low as reasonably achievable (ALARA), so as to derive maximum diagnostic information with minimum discomfort to the patient. ALARA recognizes that there will always be some radiation exposure to patients involved in radiological procedures using ionizing radiation, but it also recognizes that these exposures can be minimized.

Principles of Radiation Protection

- *Justification:* Justification of a practice, e.g. the benefit to risk ratio is high for CT brain in cerebrovascular hemorrhage and low in screening mammography in women below 35 years.
- *Optimized protection:* "Optimization of the radiological procedure" is to reduce radiation exposures to the minimum levels. This optimization is possible by good quality assurance and quality control.

- *Dose limitation:* By using high frequency generators which enable "high kV and low mAs" technique. The high kV beam has higher energy photons, which undergo a lesser degree of beam attenuation and greater penetration of the beam through the patient. Therefore the tissue deposition of photons is reduced, which reduces the radiation dose to the patient.

Triad of Radiation Protection Actions

Time

The exposure time is related to radiation exposure and exposure rate (exposure per unit time).

Exposure = Exposure rate × Time

This implies that if the exposure time is kept short, then the resulting dose to the individual is small.

Distance

Distance is between the source of radiation and the exposed individual. The exposure to the individual decreases inversely as the square of the distance. This is known as the inverse square law. Another important consideration with respect to distance relates to the source-to-image receptor distance (SID). The appropriate SIDs for various examinations must always be maintained. Long SID results in less divergent beam and thus decreases the concentration of photons in the patients. Short SID results in the reverse action and increases the patient dose. Hence the longest possible SID should be employed in examinations.

Shielding

Shielding implies that certain materials (concrete, lead) will attenuate radiation when they are placed between the source of radiation and the exposed individual.

X-ray Tube Shielding (Source Shielding)

X-ray tube housing is lined with thin sheets of lead because X-rays produced in the tube are scattered in all directions. This shielding is intended to protect both patients and personnel from leakage radiation. AERB recommends a maximum allowable leakage radiation from tube housing not greater than 1 mGy per hour per $100 \, cm^2$.

Room Shielding (Structural Shielding)

The lead lined walls of radiology department are referred to as protective barriers because they are designed to protect individuals located outside the

X-ray rooms from unwanted radiation. Primary barrier is one which is directly struck by the primary or the useful beam. Secondary barrier is one which is exposed to secondary radiation either by leakage from X-ray tube or by scattered radiation from the patient.

X-ray Examination Room

The room housing an X-ray unit is not less than 18 m^2 for general purpose radiography and conventional fluoroscopy equipment. In case the installation is located in a residential complex, it is ensured that (i) wall of the X-ray rooms on which primary X-ray beam falls is not less than 35 cm thick brick or equivalent, (ii) walls of the X-ray room on which scattered X-rays fall is not less than 23 cm thick brick or equivalent, (iii) there is a shielding equivalent to at least 23 cm thick brick or 1.7 mm lead in front of the doors and windows of the X-ray room to protect the adjacent areas, either used by general public or not under possession of the owner of the X-ray room. Unshielded openings in an X-ray room for ventilation or natural light are located above a height of 2 m from the finished level outside the X-ray room.

Patient Waiting Area

Patient waiting areas are provided outside the X-ray room. A suitable warning signal such as red light and a warning placard is provided at a conspicuous place outside the X-ray room and kept 'ON' when the unit is in use to warn persons not connected with the particular examination from entering the room.

CT Room

The highly collimated X-ray beam in CT results in markedly non uniform distribution of absorbed dose perpendicular to the tomographic plane during the CT exposure. Therefore the size of the CT room housing the gantry of the CT unit as recommended by AERB should not be less than 25 m^2. The walls and viewing window of the control booth, which should have lead equivalents of 1.5 mm. The location of control booth, which should not be located where the primary beam falls directly, and the radiation should be scattered twice before entering the booth.

Personnel Shielding

Personnel should remain in the radiation environment only when necessary. The distance between the personnel and the patient should be maximized when practical as the intensity of radiation decreases as the square of distance (inverse square law). Shielding

apparel should be used as and when necessary which comprise of lead aprons, eye glasses with side shields, hand gloves and thyroid shields.

Lead aprons are shielding apparel recommended for use by radiation workers. These are classified as a secondary barrier to the effects of ionizing radiation. These aprons protect an individual only from secondary (scattered) radiation, not the primary beam. 0.25 mm lead thickness attenuates 66% of the beam at 75 kVp and 1 mm attenuates 99% of the beam at same kVp. It is recommended that for general purpose radiography the minimum thickness of lead equivalent in the protective apparel should be 0.5 mm. When not in use, all protective apparel should be hung on properly designed racks, otherwise there can be cracks or tear in protective lead sheet. Protective apparel also should be radiographed for defects such as internal cracks and tears at least once a year. It is recommended that women radiation workers should wear a customized lead apron that reaches below mid thigh level and wraps completely around the pelvis. This would eliminate an accidental exposure to a conceptus.

Lead Free Aprons (Zero Lead Aprons)

Conventional protective aprons are heavy as they are made of lead, so the physician may not tolerate wearing one for long procedures. Lightweight alloy alternatives are a necessity as an increased number of physicians and technicians are required to wear aprons for longer time periods during more varied examinations. Nonlead protective aprons made of environment friendly, nontoxic, composite materials have been developed. Nonlead aprons consist of composite materials, mainly tungsten, bismuth, antimony and tin. They are 20% lighter than lead aprons.

Lead equivalence is measured by comparing the protection provided by pure lead sheet against that provided by the protective apron. Zero lead aprons refers to lead free apron.

Sievert

Sievert (Sv) is a unit used to derive a quantity called equivalent dose. This relates the absorbed dose in human tissue to the effective biological damage of the radiation. Equivalent dose is often expressed in terms of millionth of a sievert, or micro-sievert (µSv). To determine equivalent dose (Sv), you multiply absorbed dose (Gy) by a quality factor (Q) that is unique to the type of incident radiation. One sievert is equivalent to 100 rem.

$\quad$ 1 Sv = 10,00,000 µSv

$\quad$ mSv = 1,000 µSv

Pregnant Radiation Worker

The NCRP (National Council on Radiological Protection and measurements) recommends that the dose to the fetus in *pregnant radiation worker* should not exceed 0.5 mSv per month. The ICRP recommends that the total dose to the abdomen of the mother should not exceed 2 mSv during entire pregnancy.

Ten day rule: All females of reproductive age who need an X-ray examination should get it done within first 10 days of menstrual cycle to avoid irradiation of possible conception.

Radiography of area remote from fetus can be done safely at any time during pregnancy also by using protective lead apron, covering the fetus.

FILM BADGE

The film badge dosimeter, or film badge, is a *dosimeter* used for monitoring cumulative *exposure* to *ionizing radiation*. The badge consists of two parts: *photographic film* and a holder. The film is removed and *developed* to measure exposure. The film badge is used to measure and record radiation exposure due to gamma rays, X-rays and beta particles. The film is packaged in a light proof, vapor proof envelope preventing light, moisture or chemical vapors from affecting the film. A special film is used which is coated with two different emulsions. One side is coated with a large grain, fast emulsion that is sensitive to low levels of exposure. The other side of the film is coated with a fine grain, slow emulsion that is less sensitive to exposure. The combination of a low-sensitivity and high sensitivity *emulsion* extends the *dynamic range* to several orders of magnitude. The film is backed by a sheet of lead foil to absorb radiation from behind the badge. The film is contained inside a film holder or badge. The badge incorporates a series of filters to determine the quality of the radiation. To monitor *gamma rays* or *x-rays*, the filters are *metal*, usually *tin* or *lead*. To monitor *beta particle emission*, the filters use various densities of *plastic*. The badge holder also contains an open window to determine radiation exposure due to beta particles. Beta particles are effectively shielded by a thin amount of material. The major advantages of a film badge as a personnel monitoring device are that it provides a permanent record, it is able to distinguish between different energies of photons, and it can measure doses due to different types of radiation. It is quite accurate for exposures greater than 100 mrem (millirem). The major disadvantages are that it must be developed and read by a processor (which is time consuming), prolonged heat exposure can affect the film, and exposures of less than 20 millirem of gamma radiation cannot be accurately measured. Film badges

Table 8.1 Dose limits

	Occupational	Public
Effective dose	20 mSv/year averaged*	1 mSv in a year over 5 years
Annual equivalent dose to		
Lens of eye	150 mSv	15 mSv
Skin	500 mSv	50 mSv
Hands and Feet	500 mSv	50 mSv

*With further provision that dose in any single year > 30 mSv.

Table 8.2 Average effective dose involved in various modalities

Modality	Average effective dose in mSv
X-ray chest	0.02
X-ray skull	0.03
X-ray spine	0.4
IVP	2
Barium	2–7
CT head	2
CT chest	8
CT abdomen/Pelvis	10

need to be worn correctly so that the dose they receive accurately represents the dose the wearer receives. Whole body badges are worn on the body between the neck and the waist, often on the belt or a shirt pocket. Pregnant women should wear a second badge over abdomen beneath the leaded apron. The clip-on badge is worn most often when performing X-ray or gamma radiography. Usually the badges are returned after one month and dosimetric comparison is made with standard films exposed to known amounts of radiation. Dose limits for occupational and public is displayed in Table 8.1 and the average effective dose involved in various imaging modalities is exhibited in Table 8.2.

Thermoluminescent Dosimeter TLD BADGES

A TLD (Thermoluminescence dosimeter) measures *ionizing radiation* exposure by measuring the amount of visible light emitted from crystal in the detector when the crystal is heated. The amount of light emitted is dependent upon the radiation exposure. Materials exhibiting thermoluminescence in response to ionizing radiation include *calcium fluoride* (CaF_2), *lithium fluoride* (LiF), *calcium sulfate* ($CaSO_4$), *lithium borate* ($Li_2B_4O_7$), *calcium borate, potassium bromide* and *feldspar*. When a TLD is exposed to ionizing radiation at ambient temperatures, the radiation interacts with the phosphor crystal and deposits all or part of the incident energy in that material. Some of the atoms in the material that absorb that energy become ionized, producing free electrons and areas lacking one or more electrons, called holes. Imperfections in the crystal lattice structure act as sites where free electrons can become trapped and locked into place.

Heating the crystal causes the crystal lattice to vibrate, releasing the trapped electrons in the process. Released electrons return to the original ground state, releasing the captured energy from ionization as light, hence the name thermo luminescent. Released light is counted using photomultiplier tubes and the number of photons counted is proportional to the quantity of radiation striking the phosphor.

TLD are often used instead of the film badge. Like a film badge, it is worn for a period of time (usually 3 months or less) and then must be processed to determine the dose received, if any. Thermoluminescent dosimeters can measure doses as low as 1 mrem. The advantages of a TLD over other personnel monitors are its linearity of response to dose, its relative energy independence, and its sensitivity to low doses. It is also reusable, which is an advantage over film badges. However, no permanent record or re-readability is provided and an immediate, on the job readout is not possible.

Patient Shielding

Thyroid, breast and gonads are shielded to protect these organs, especially in children and young adults. In gonad shielding, a lead apron is placed appropriately on the patient to protect the gonads from primary beam radiation exposure. A lead bib and collar worn over the patient's neck and thorax have been documented to effectively shield radiosensitive organs like the thyroid and the breast, and are therefore recommended for routine use in dental X-rays and head CT examinations.

Radiation Protection Survey and Program

The hospital administration/owner of the X-ray facility is expected to appoint a Radiation Safety Committee (RSC), and a Radiation Safety Officer (RSO).

This survey has 5 phases
1. *Investigation:* To obtain information regarding layout of the department, workload, personnel monitoring and records.
2. *Inspection:* Each diagnostic installation in the department is examined for its protection status with respect to its operating factors, control booth and availability of protection devices.
3. *Measurement:* Measurements are conducted on exposure factors. In addition scattered radiation and patient dose measurements in radiography and fluoroscopy are performed.
4. *Evaluation:* The radiation protection status of the department is evaluated by examination of records, equipment working, status of protective clothing and the radiation doses obtained from phase-3.
5. *Recommendations:* A report is prepared on the protection status of the department and the problem areas if any identified, for which recommendations are made regarding corrective measures.

Radiation Safety Officer

Radiation safety officer (RSO) should be an individual with extensive training and education in areas such as radiation protection, radiation physics, radiation biology, instrumentation, dosimetry and shielding design. AERB has specified duties of the RSO which include assisting the employer in meeting the relevant regulatory requirements applicable to his/her X-ray installation. He/she shall implement all radiation surveillance measures, conduct periodic radiation protection surveys, maintain proper records of periodic quality assurance tests, and personnel doses, instruct all workers on relevant safety measures, educate and train new entrants, and take local measures. The RSO should also ensure that all radiation measuring and monitoring instruments in his/her custody are properly calibrated and maintained in good condition.

Optimization of protection can be achieved by optimizing the procedure to administer a radiation dose which is as low as reasonably achievable (ALARA), so as to derive maximum diagnostic information with minimum discomfort to the patient.

9

Ultrasound Physics

Anand Kamat

Sound is a mechanical form of energy, which travels through a medium as a wave, producing alternate compression and rarefaction. The audible range of sound energy by human beings is from 20 Hz to 20000 Hz. Ultrasound is defined as sound having frequencies above audible range. The frequencies applied for diagnostic ultrasound are from 2 MHz (megahertz) to 15 MHz.

The number of complete cycles of sound per second is called the frequency of ultrasound. The frequency is denoted by 'ʋ'. The distance between two successive rarefactions or compressions is called as the wavelength (Fig. 9.1) of the sound. It is denoted by Greek letter 'λ'.

VELOCITY OF PROPAGATION

Formula: velocity v = frequency ʋ × wavelength λ. The resistance of the medium to compression force produced by sound energy determines the velocity of propagation in that medium. Density of medium is inversely proportional and stiffness of medium is directly proportional to v, the velocity. The propagation velocity of ultrasound is assumed by the machine to be 1540 m/sec, in all body tissues. However, it actually varies from this figure from tissue to tissue. This can sometimes give rise to false distance measurements.

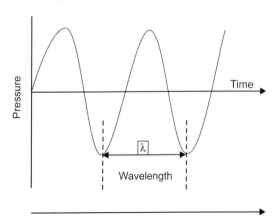

Fig. 9.1 Sound wave propagation

MEASUREMENT OF DISTANCE BY MACHINE

The distance of a reflecting surface from the ultrasound probe can be calculated by the machine provided the propagation velocity of sound for that tissue is known. As it is assumed to be 1540 m/sec, the distance of a reflecting interface when an ultrasound pulse is sent into the body and the time taken for that echo to return is measured, it is possible to calculate the depth of that interface from the transducer. This is then displayed on the machine screen.

ACOUSTIC IMPEDANCE

Formula is Z = ρv, where v is the velocity of ultrasound in that medium and ρ (ρ = Rho, it is the 17th letter of the Greek alphabet) is the density of the medium through which ultrasound is travelling. There are different interfaces in the body, e.g. fat and air, urine in bladder and bladder wall, liver tissue and vessel etc. Ultrasound machines work on the principle of detection of reflected echo and the reflected echo at any interface is directly proportional to the difference between the acoustic impedances of those two tissues forming that interface. Larger part of ultrasound is reflected when difference in acoustic impedances is more and smaller part of ultrasound is reflected when difference in acoustic impedances is small. When a material is without any interface, e.g. urine in bladder, no ultrasound will be reflected from points within such a region.

REFLECTION

Reflection (Fig. 9.2) can be either diffuse reflection or specular reflection. A diffuse reflection of ultrasound takes place in many solid tissue organs in the body e.g. liver, spleen. Here the insonated ultrasound is reflected in multiple directions from that point and the part that is reflected in the direction of transducer will contribute to the image. Specular reflection takes place when angle of incidence of ultrasound is equal

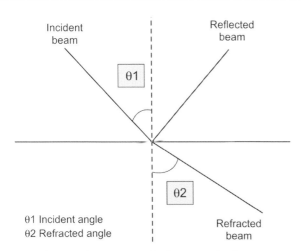

θ1 Incident angle
θ2 Refracted angle

Fig. 9.2 Phenomenon of reflection and refraction

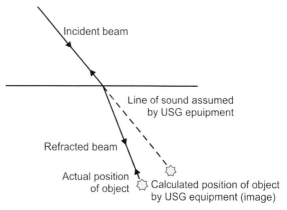

Fig. 9.3 Refraction artifact

to angle of reflection of ultrasound. This requires a smooth type of reflector, e.g. wall of an artery, wall of a vein, capsule of liver or dome of diaphragm. These are termed as specular reflectors. Obviously these reflectors will reflect ultrasound back to transducer only if direction of beam is perpendicular to the interface. Reflection co-efficient (R) is the ratio of the intensity of the reflected wave to the incident wave.

Reflection coefficient R = $(Z1 - Z2)^2 / (Z1 + Z2)^2$.

REFRACTION

When ultrasound crosses an interface, it changes its direction and this phenomenon is called as refraction (Fig. 9.3). The terms of physics to be used here are angle of incidence and angle of refraction. However computer does not understand this, which leads to an artifact as the reflected echo from a structure beyond this refracting interface will be placed in image at a different depth and at a different direction.

$$\text{Snell's law: } \frac{v1}{v2} = \frac{\sin\theta 1}{\sin\theta 2}$$

v1 - velocity in medium 1
v2 - velocity in medium 2
θ1 - angle of incidence
θ2 - angle of refraction

ATTENUATION

As ultrasound passes through a body tissue, there occurs a gradual loss in its intensity and power. This is called attenuation of ultrasound by body tissues. There are multiple factors causing such attenuation. Ultimately the absorbed sound energy produces heat energy in the tissues, thus there is conversion of one form of energy into another form of energy. If frequency of transducer is more, attenuation takes place fast in the

tissues. If frequency of transducer is less, attenuation takes place slow in the tissues. Therefore a probe of 3.5 MHz will have greater depth of image than a probe of 5 MHz. Time gain compensation (TGC) is therefore required to produce an image of uniform brightness on monitor. TGC augments the reflected echoes from deeper regions because these signals are weak due to attenuation.

Sound power is measured in decibels and it is a relative term. Hence attenuation is measured in decibels.

Decibel = log of sound power 1/log of sound power 2
Intensity of sound I = power in Watts/Area in cm^2

ULTRASOUND TRANSDUCER

Transducer sends ultrasound into body of patient and also receives the ultrasound that is sent back from body tissues after reflection which will go to form image. Ultrasound is produced by piezoelectric effect Transducer incorporates a piezoelectric element, which converts electrical signals into mechanical vibrations (transmit mode) and mechanical vibrations (Fig. 9.4) into electrical signals (receive mode). Many factors, including material, mechanical and electrical construction, and the external mechanical and electrical load conditions, influence the behavior of a transducer. Mechanical construction includes parameters such as the radiation surface area, mechanical damping, housing, connector type and other variables of physical construction.

Piezoelectric effect and piezoelectric material: Some substances change shape when electric potential is applied to them and come back to original form when electric potential is stopped. If this is done very rapidly they will go in vibration and emit ultrasound. This property is called piezoelectric effect and these materials are called as piezoelectric materials. Also when they are hit by sound, they change shape and produce an electric potential at their ends.

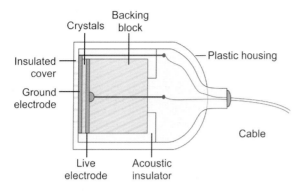

Fig. 9.4 Ultrasound transducer

Bandwidth: Multiple frequencies are produced when piezoelectric material is vibrating to produce ultrasound and this range of frequencies emitted is termed bandwidth. Bandwidth can be narrow or broad. Generally a broad bandwidth is used in present technology.

Continuous Wave (CW): Here the transducer sends continuous ultrasound energy into tissues. Here there is no time gap. This is used in Doppler studies.

Pulsed Wave (PW): Here ultrasound that is emitted by the transducer is in the form of multiple pulses. These pulses are of same intensity and are spaced by time gaps.

Pulse repetition frequency (PRF): PRF is the number of pulses generated in one second. This term PRF is very commonly used in diagnostic ultrasound. The time gap between the two pulses is such that the reflected echo of earlier pulse reaches the transducer before the next pulse is sent.

Pulse length: Each pulse contains a certain number of cycles and thus pulse length PL = wavelength (λ) x number of cycles in that pulse. Certain damping materials are placed behind the piezoelectric material to minimize the pulse length.

Time gain compensation (TGC): We have seen that as ultrasound passes through tissues in the body, it is attenuated. As a result reflected echoes start becoming weaker and weaker as ultrasound goes deeper and deeper in the tissues. If image is produced without any processing, it will be very bright for the superficial tissues and dim for the deeper tissues. To avoid this, reflected echoes from deeper tissues are augmented in such a way that an image of uniform brightness is produced on the monitor this is called TGC. This control is operated by the operator and is a very important control of the machine. Being manually operated control of the machine is operator dependent.

Dynamic range: Monitor shows this in decibels and it is the ratio of highest to lowest of ultrasound intensities that can be displayed.

Gel: Gel is placed between transducer and patient's body so that maximum energy goes into patient's body. This removes minute air gaps between transducer and body surface. Major components of ultrasound gel are propylene glycol, glycerin, phenoxyethanol.

PRESENTATION OF ULTRASOUND IMAGE ON MONITOR

A mode: This is shown as a wave on oscilloscope. The height of this wave is proportional to the amplitude of the retuning echo. This is mostly not in use except some ophthalmic centers for the eye ball.

M mode: Motion mode is plotted against time graph. This image presents motion of structures in a single line below the transducer in any tissue. This is mainly used in adult or fetal heart studies, called as echocardiography. This is useful in studying valve and wall motions in time axis.

B mode: This is the most commonly used format of image presentation. It is almost always done in real time to show movements of structures below probe, e.g. diaphragm, peristalsis, etc. Here brighter part means tissue is more reflective and darker part means tissue is less reflective. This range from dark to white with many intermediate shades is called gray scale.

Pixels and monitor: Pixel is the smallest unit in a monitor representing a reflected signal in gray scale. Each pixel is capable of showing on monitor 256 grades of gray scale image intensities. Thus different tissues having different echogenecities can be finely differentiated. The total number of pixels used depends upon the format of the monitor. The commonly used formats are 512 × 640 and 512 × 512.

Frame rate: As transducer moves, different planes of body come under it. When they are displayed at more than 16 frames per second, the human brain appreciates it as a continuous movement and not as subsequent frames. Commonly 16 to 60 frames per second are used. Thus moving diaphragm, peristalsis, respiratory movements of liver and spleen, fetal and adult heart movements can be appreciated in real time. This is an important aspect for making diagnosis.

Transducers: These can be mechanical type or electronic type. Now mostly electronic type is used. Mechanical sector probe, used previously, used a moving transducer to produce a sector format of image.

Linear array: Mainly used for superficial parts, e.g. thyroid, testes, arteries and veins, etc. In this the transducer elements are placed along a single line (Fig. 9.5). Each element will image a solid rectangle of tissue below it. The ultrasound beam from these elements goes perpendicular to the probe. Hence a

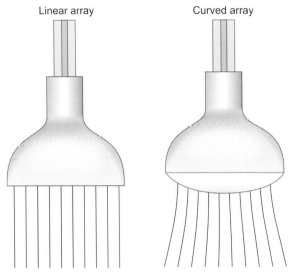

Linear array   Curved array

Fig. 9.5 Types of transducers

rectangular image is produced. It is possible to focus at a particular depth.

Phased array: Here the arrangement of the piezo-electric elements is same as that of a linear array, i.e. they are arranged in a linear fashion. However these elements are activated in a particular exact sequence and this leads to a beam that is rapidly undulating, thus ultimately producing a sector type of beam and a sector type of image format. These are useful when window of access is small, e.g. intercostals space.

Curved array: Here the piezoelectric elements are placed in one curved line (Fig. 9.5), thus producing a sector type of beam and a sector type of image format.

Annular array: Here the piezoelectric elements are placed in concentric circles or in a rectangle like matrix format. This type of arrangement produces a superior type of focusing and also a superior type of resolution. They are used in 3D data acquisition.

Scanning by Compounding: Many image degrading artifacts are dependent on the angle of scanning. Thus artifacts produced while scanning in one angle are not produced while scanning in another angle. In this technique same structure is scanned at two or more different angles, and then summation is done of images. This eliminates some noise and improves the image quality. This can be mainly used to image superficial structures as angle changing is possible. This method in termed as spatial compound scanning.

Currently, 4D ultrasound is extensively used in the field of obstetrics, interventional radiology and in fetal medicine during the procedure.

The quality of image depends upon resolution. The closest distance between any two reflectors that will produce two distinctly separate images is called the resolution. Resolutions can be:

Axial: Resolution which is along the path of ultrasound beam. This depends upon the pulse length. Pulse length reduces as frequency increases. Hence it is directly related to the frequency. Hence high frequency probes will lead to more axial resolution.

Lateral: Resolution in a direction that is perpendicular to the direction of ultrasound beam and which lies in the plane of image is called lateral resolution.

Azimuth: Resolution in a plane which is perpendicular to the direction of ultrasound beam as well as to the probe is called azimuth resolution. Also called elevation resolution and this is related to the thickness of the beam.

10

Doppler

Santosh Konde

Doppler methods are unique and important among ultrasound imaging techniques in that they have the potential to offer information related to the blood supply of an organ rather than its morphology, although, they also derive information from the interaction of a ultrasound beam with body part being examined. The Doppler Effect was named after Johann Christian Doppler (1803–1853), an Austrian mathematician and physicist, who theorized that sound waves from a moving source would be closer together as the sound source came closer, and further apart as the sound source went further away. The Doppler Effect is explained as the change in frequency and wavelength of a wave which results from a source moving with respect to the medium, a receiver moving with respect to the medium, or even a moving medium. The Doppler effect is applicable to any kind of wave, whether electromagnetic like light or mechanical like ultrasound.

In ultrasound, the Doppler effect is used to measure blood flow velocity where the reflector is the red blood cell. Ultrasound reflected from red blood cells will change in frequency according to the blood flow velocity. When the direction of blood flow is towards the Doppler transducer, the echoes from blood reflected back to the transducer will have a higher frequency than the one emitted from the transducer. When the direction is away from the transducer, the echoes will have a lower frequency than those emitted by the transducer. The difference in frequency between transmitted and received echoes is called the Doppler frequency shift, and this shift in frequency is directly proportional to the blood flow velocity. Thus, the basis of Doppler ultrasonography is the fact that reflected ultrasonic waves from a moving interface will undergo a frequency shift proportional to the velocity of the reflecting interface.

Doppler equation: The change in frequency is directly proportional to the velocity of the moving target and can be calculated using the Doppler equation. The Doppler equation describes the relationship of the Doppler frequency shift to target velocity.

Doppler equation: $\Delta F = F_R - F_T = 2F_T V \cos \theta / C$

Where, ΔF = the Doppler frequency shift, F_R = reflected frequency, F_T = transmitted frequency, V = the velocity of the moving object, θ = the angle between velocity of moving object and line joining object and transducer, C = velocity of sound in that medium.

The frequency difference is equal to the reflected frequency (F_R) minus the transmitted frequency (F_T). If the reflected frequency is higher, then there is a positive Doppler shift and the object is moving toward the transducer, but if the reflected frequency is lower, there is a negative Doppler shift and the object is moving away from the transducer (Fig. 10.1).

In ideal situation the Doppler shift would be calculated as if the ultrasound was parallel to the target's direction. However, this seldom occurs in clinical practice, because the transducer is rarely pointed, but parallel to the length of a blood vessel. In clinical practice, the ultrasound waves would approach the target at an angle, called the Doppler angle.

Doppler angle: The Doppler angle (θ) is the angle of insonation. Estimation of target velocity requires

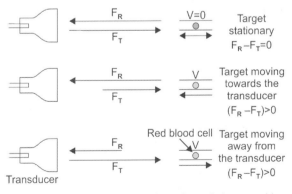

Fig. 10.1 On stationary target the reflected ultrasound has the same frequency as the transmitted sound, so transmitted (FT) and reflected (FR) frequencies are same. However, in moving target there is a change in the frequency of the sound reflected from the target interface.

Abbreviations: F_R = Reflected frequency, F_T = Transmitted frequency.

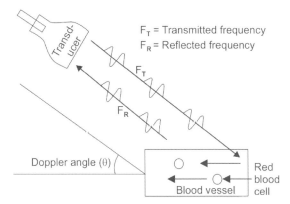

F_T = Transmitted frequency
F_R = Reflected frequency

Fig. 10.2 The ultrasound beam strikes the moving target at an angle referred as Doppler angle (θ) which reduces the frequency shift in proportion to the cosine of this angle. The Doppler angle gives corrected flow velocity

precise measurements of both the Doppler frequency shift and the angle of insonation to the direction of the velocity of estimated target. If the Doppler angle can be measured, flow velocity can be estimated by angle correction, which involves aligning an indicator on the duplex image along the longitudinal axis of the vessel (Fig. 10.2).

As seen in the Doppler equation, the dependence on the Doppler angle is in the form of a cosine which gives the component of the flow velocity vector that is parallel to the sound beam. If the direction of sound propagation is directly opposite to the flow direction ($\theta = 0$), the maximum positive Doppler shift is obtained. If the angle between these two directions is non-zero, lesser Doppler shifts will occur. Because, the error in the estimation of Doppler angle is more at large angles and Doppler shifts become very small at large angles, Doppler measurements are not reliably achieved at Doppler angles greater than 60 to 70°. The cosine of 90° is zero, so if the ultrasound beam is perpendicular to the direction of blood flow, there will be no Doppler shift appearing as if there is no flow in the vessel. Therefore, the angle of insonation should also be less than 60° at all times, since the cosine function has a steeper curve above this angle magnifying the errors in angle correction.

The Doppler shift measured by a Doppler ultrasonography is proportional to the operating frequency of the instrument. Higher frequency instruments provide higher Doppler shifts as higher ultrasound frequencies are reflected more strongly while lower are reflected less strongly. However, attenuation of the ultrasound in tissues increases with frequency. The attenuation has the dominant effect so that higher frequencies do not penetrate as effectively as lower ones. The frequencies comparable to that used for sonography are used for Doppler measurements, i.e. 2 to 10 MHz. Because many abdominal vessels

lie several centimeters beneath the surface, Doppler frequencies in the range of 3 to 3.5 MHz are usually required for abdominal Doppler. In practice Doppler frequencies for given depth applications are slightly less than the frequency used for imaging at that depth. *Doppler signal processing and display:* Several options exist for the processing of the Doppler shift, to provide useful information regarding the direction and velocity of blood. All Doppler techniques display flow information, but some are optimized to display certain characteristics of blood flow. For example, conventional Doppler imaging produces a wave form that can be used to calculate the actual flow rate in a vessel, whereas color flow Doppler displays the same information by superimposing the image of moving blood in color on the usual gray scale real time image. The color flow highlights the areas of high flow and disturbed flow, which can then be examined more thoroughly and quantitatively with conventional duplex Doppler imaging. Doppler frequency shifts in most clinical situations are audible to the human ear and may be analyzed by ear with training. More commonly the Doppler shift data are displayed in graphic form as a frequency spectrum of the returning signal over time. These frequencies are analyzed using spectral analysis, which separates the signal into individual components and assigns a relative importance. Fast Fourier transformation is the most popular method of spectral analysis. The envelope of the spectrum represents the maximum frequencies present at any given point of time, and the width of the spectrum at any point indicates the range of the frequencies present. The presence of large number of frequencies at a given point results in spectral broadening.

Continuous wave (CW) Doppler: The simplest Doppler devices use continuous wave ultrasound using dual element transducer that transmit and receive ultrasound continuously. The transmit and receive beams overlap in a Doppler sample volume some distance from the transducer face. There is continuous transducer transmission and reception; echoes from all depths within the area arrive at the transducer simultaneously. Although direction of flow can be determined with CW Doppler, these devices do not allow discrimination of motion coming from various depths. These are primarily used at the bedside to confirm blood flow in superficial vessels, as they are good at detecting low velocities.

Pulsed wave (PW) Doppler: Pulsed wave Doppler devices have single element transducer which emits brief pulses of ultrasound energy. The time interval between transmitting and then receiving the reflected sound can be used to calculate the depth from where the Doppler shift arises and time-based gating of the receiving channel allows the definition of a fixed measuring distance referred to as the Sample volume or Doppler gate. The Doppler sample volume can be chosen as to shape, depth, and position in sampling the flow data. For example, the depth is chosen by processing only the signals that return to the transducer in a stipulated time. The number of pulses transmitted by the system within a second is referred to as the pulse repetition frequency (PRF). The greater the sample-volume depth, the longer the time before the echoes are returned, and the longer the delay between pulse transmission with lower maximum PRF setting.

Duplex scanning: PW Doppler combined with 2D, real-time, B-mode scanner is known as a Duplex scanner. The term duplex scanning was first coined by F.E. Barber in 1974, when he described how he had combined B-mode ultrasound with pulsed wave Doppler. Using a multigated system, the Doppler signals produce a two-dimensional image and the Doppler image is superimposed on the B-mode image producing a duplex image. The B-mode image allows the precise position and control of the Doppler sample volume.

Color flow Doppler imaging: This is the most common form of Doppler used in diagnostic Radiology. In color flow Doppler imaging systems, the velocity of the flow is displayed in the image as a color flow map by color encoding the Doppler frequency shift. The reflected signals from red blood cells are displayed in color as a function of their motion towards or away from the transducer and are superimposed on the B-Mode anatomic grayscale image. The degree of the shade of the color reflects the blood flow velocity. The use of color shades to display variations of Doppler shift frequency allows a semiquantitative estimate of flow, to be made from the image alone. The display of flow throughout the image field allows the position and the orientation of the vessel of interest to be observed at all times. Flow within the vessel is observed at all points and the stenotic jets and focal areas of turbulence are displayed that might be overlooked with duplex instrumentations only. Color flow Doppler imaging helps in accurate determination of flow direction. Color flow mapping allows visualization of small vessels that are difficult to assess using other imaging methods like duplex alone.

Power Mode Doppler: Power Doppler is the use of a color map that displays the integrated power of the Doppler signal (amplitude) instead of its mean frequency shift. The displayed color map shows the distribution of the amplitude. The image does not provide any information related to flow direction or flow velocity. Power Doppler is most commonly used to evaluate blood flow through vessels within solid organs. As there is no aliasing, power Doppler gives increased sensitivity to flow detection and is up to five times more sensitive at detecting blood flow than color Doppler.

Interpretation of Doppler signal: Doppler ultrasound makes it possible to identify vessel, determine the direction of blood flow, and evaluate narrowing or occlusion, and characterize flow to organs and tumors. Doppler data components that must be evaluated both in spectral display and in color flow imaging include the Doppler shift frequency and amplitude, the Doppler angle, the spatial distribution of frequencies across the vessel and the temporal variation of the signal. The sign of frequency shift (positive or negative) indicates the direction of flow relative to the transducer.

Doppler waveforms and indices: Doppler waveforms are tracings of the relationship of the velocity of the blood flowing in a vessel over time. The velocity is determined from the Doppler shift frequency. The high-resistance arterial waveform shows a rapid fall in velocity following systole (Fig. 10.3A). The characteristic normal peripheral arterial waveform has a high velocity forward flow component during systole (ventricular contraction), followed by a brief reversal of flow in early diastole, due to peripheral resistance, ending with a low velocity forward flow phase in late diastole, caused by the recoil of the vessel wall. A low-resistance artery, such as the renal artery, shows continuous flow during diastole (Fig. 10.3B). A low-resistance vein, such as the portal vein typically shows low velocity and low resistance waveform (Fig. 10.3C). Information related to the resistance to flow in the distal vascular tree can be obtained by the analysis of changes of blood velocity with time shown in the Doppler spectral display (Figs 10.4A and B). Vessel stenosis is typically associated with large Doppler frequency shifts in both systole and diastole at the site of greatest narrowing, with turbulent flow in poststenotic segment. In peripheral vessels, analysis of Doppler changes allows accurate prediction of the degree of vessel narrowing.

Systole -"S" the maximum amplitude representing the peak systolic velocity (PSV)

Diastole -"D" the slowest forward flow representing end diastolic velocity (EDV)

The resistive index (RI) = (S-D)/S, The higher the resistance, the higher the resistive index

Systolic/Diastolic ratio (S/D ratio) = S/D

Pulsatility index (PI) = (S-D)/M, where M is mean velocity.

Negative velocity represents flow away from the transducer, as can be seen where the waveform falls below the axis between systole and diastole.

Wall filters: Doppler instruments detect motion not only from blood flow but also from adjacent structures. Wall filter is a necessary device that eliminates

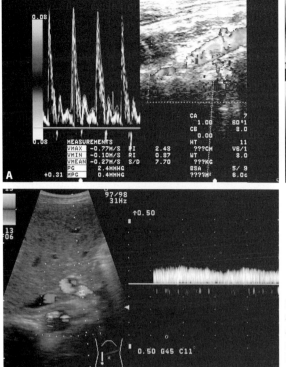

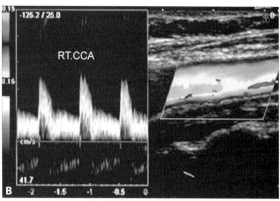

Figs 10.3A to C The high-resistance arterial waveform shows a rapid fall in velocity following systole (A), low-resistance arterial waveform shows continuous flow during diastole (B), low-resistance vein, such as the portal vein typically shows low velocity and low resistance waveform (C) (*For color version, see Plate 1*)

low frequency signals from the Doppler spectrum waveform, which are usually produced by low velocity structures such as vessel walls and tissues next to vessels (Fig. 10.5). Wall filters are designed as High Pass Filters that remove low frequencies, which fall below a certain frequency cutoff point. The Wall Filter setting is variable and can be adjusted by the user. These filters may also remove genuine signals from low velocity blood flow like low velocity venous or diastolic flow. In certain clinical situations, the measurement of these slower flow velocities is of clinical importance, and the improper selection of wall filters may result in serious errors of interpretations. To prevent these errors, the wall filter should be set to the lowest practical level.

Spectral broadening: Blood flow in vessels does not flow at uniform velocities and spectral broadening occurs due to mixture of large number of different velocities in a sample volume (Fig. 10.6). It refers to presence of a large range of flow velocities at a given point in the pulse cycle and are important criteria of high grade vessel narrowing. It may also be produced by the selection of an excessively large sample volume or by the placement of the sample volume near the vessel wall.

The Nyquist Limit and Aliasing: PW Doppler gives an accurate measure of the blood flow at a specific area and allows the detection of both velocity and direction. The reception of the returning signals is timed,

and shows flows at specific depths. To ensure that samples from only selected depth are analyzed when using pulsed wave, it is necessary to wait for the echo from the area of interest to reach transducer before transmitting the next pulse. This limits pulse repetition frequency (PRF), a lower PRF being required for greater depths. The highest velocity accurately measured is called the Nyquist limit. Errors in the accuracy of the information arise if the velocities exceed a certain speed of the Nyquist limits. The Nyquist limit states that the sampling frequency must be greater than twice the highest frequency of the received signal for accurate sampling and measurements. The Nyquist limit is defined as being half the PRF. If the PRF is less than twice the maximum frequency shift produced by movement of target (the Nyquist limit), the resulting data will contain artifacts known as aliasing. Color flow Doppler utilizes this effect allowing the detection of flow disturbances from laminar to turbulent flow (Fig. 10.7A). Depending on the degree of aliasing, the high frequencies "wrap around" and are displayed on the opposite side of the baseline, so that blood appears to be flowing in the opposite direction (Fig. 10.7B). Aliasing can be reduced by increasing the PRF, repositioning the baseline, increasing the Doppler angle, or by using lower frequency transducer.

Sample volume size: Sample volume is an area in 2D image from which Doppler signals on being acquired

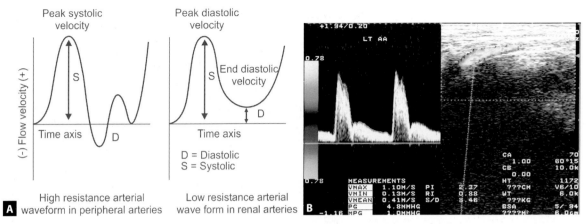

Figs 10.4A and B (A) Graphical Doppler spectral display; (B) Typical spectral waveform pattern with parameter display (*For color version, see Plate 1*)

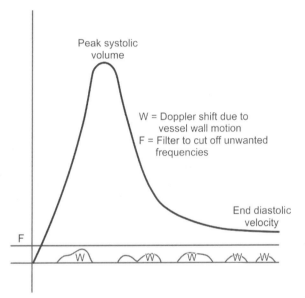

Fig. 10.5 Doppler frequency shift

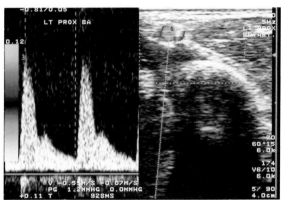

Fig. 10.6 Spectral broadening occurs due to mixture of large number of different velocities in a sample volume with filling—in of the "window" under the spectral curve (*For color version, see Plate 2*)

for spectral display using Doppler instruments, motion is detected not only from blood flow in vessels, but also from adjacent structures, such as the vessel walls. With pulsed wave Doppler systems, the length of Doppler sample volume can be controlled by the operator to exclude the unwanted signals from as near the vessel walls as possible and the width is determined by beam profile. The sample volume is adjusted to exclude as much of the unwanted clutter from near the vessel walls as possible.

Bio-effects of Doppler, Doppler heating and 'ALARA' principle: With B-mode imaging the number of ultrasound pulses arriving at a given point in patient over a given interval of time is relatively small and relatively little energy is deposited at any given location. However, in spectral Doppler, multiple ultrasound pulses are sent in repetition along a line to collect the Doppler data. This results in considerably greater potential for heating than in imaging modes. Longer pulse durations are used in Doppler than with B-imaging modes. Longer pulse duration and higher PRF result in increasing the amount of energy introduced in scanning. Operator needs to be aware that switching from a B-mode imaging to Doppler mode increases the exposure conditions and the potential for bio-effects. At least some of these instruments are capable of producing temperature rise of greater than one degree, if the focal zone of the transducer is held stationary for longer time. Therefore, while using Doppler, ALARA (as low as reasonably possible) principle should be used. The physical effects of ultrasound can be divided into two groups, thermal and nonthermal.

Thermal effects: As ultrasound propagates through body, energy is lost through attenuation, along the propagation path of ultrasound by absorption. Absorption is the conversion of ultrasound energy into heat. This heat is calculated as thermal index (TI). TI = Wo/Wdeg, where Wo is the ultrasonic source

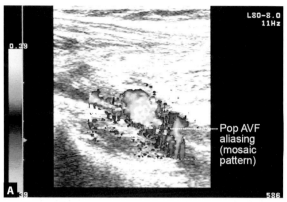
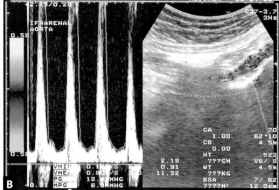

Figs 10.7A and B (A) Popliteal arteriovenous fistula (Pop AVF)-aliasing is seen because of the high velocities and Doppler shift frequencies are above the Nyquist limit. Aliasing is seen as a color change from red through yellow, to blue giving 'mosaic pattern' on color flow imaging; (B) Aortic stenosis- In Doppler waveform the peak velocity is cut off and the high frequencies "wrap around" and are displayed on the opposite side of the baseline (*For color version, see Plate 2*)

power in watts, being used in current exam, Wdeg is the ultrasonic source power, calculated as capable of producing a one degree centigrade temperature elevation under specific conditions in tissue examined.

Mechanical index (MI) reflects energy to which a target is exposed in an ultrasound beam. The mechanical index MI is the peak rarefaction pressure divided by the square root of the ultrasound frequency. It is defined for the focus of the ultrasound beam and it lessens with increasing depth.

$$MI = \frac{\text{Peak negative pressure}}{\text{square root of frequency}}$$

In clinical ultrasound systems this index usually lies between 0.1 and 0.2. In ultrasound machines, on screen display of TI and MI is provided to the operator.

Ultrasound contrast media: Ultrasound contrast media, or echo enhancers, are intravascular agents that enhance the reflection of ultrasound signals by the flowing blood for a short period after intravenous administration. These are microbubbles that are introduced in body intravenously and as they circulate through the tissue, they enhance the returning echo both in gray scale and Doppler imaging. One of the major aims in using ultrasound contrast agent in abdominal organ is to detect flow in the circulation at a flow velocity that is lower than detected by Doppler. Ultrasound contrast media act by enhancing the echogenicity of the solid components in flowing blood and by increasing the proportion of scattered and reflected ultrasound pulses, thereby improving the Doppler signal and the signal to-noise ratio. Most echo enhancers consist of gas-filled microbubbles that improve sound backscatter as a result of the large difference in acoustic impedance that exists between the gas and the liquid blood. The extent of backscatter

depends on the microbubble concentration and the reflection capacity of the individual bubbles. This capacity is a function of the scatter cross-section of the bubbles. The maximum bubble size is limited by the fact that they must pass the lungs (bubble size less than 8 μm). Short pulses of high energy can be applied to make the microbubbles burst, producing ultrasound signals that can be detected with a high degree of sensitivity. The behavior of bubbles in an acoustic field depends upon the intensity of the transmitted ultrasound beam which is monitored by means of the MI displayed by the scanner. At very low MI, the bubbles act as simple, but powerful echo enhancer which is most useful for spectral and color Doppler enhancement, but is rarely used in the liver. At slightly higher intensities the bubbles emit harmonics as they undergo nonlinear oscillations. These harmonics can be detected by harmonic and pulse inversion imaging, which form the basis of real time B mode imaging of vascular structures in the liver. Finally at the higher intensity setting of the machine used in routine scanning, the bubbles can be disrupted deliberately, emitting a strong transient echo. Detecting this echo with harmonic power Doppler remains the most sensitive means to image bubbles at very low concentrations.

Free gas bubbles: They are no more used as they cannot pass through pulmonary circulation.

Encapsulated air bubbles: The example is Levovist which is a dry mixture comprising 99.9% microcrystalline galactose microparticles and 1% palmitic acid. On disolution in sterile water, 3 to 5 micromilimeter sized microbubbles are formed. The microbubbles are stabilized as they get coated with palmitic acid, which also slows their dissolution. These microbubbles are highly echogenic and are capable of transit through pulmonary circuit.

Low solubility gas bubbles: The shells that stabilize these types of microbubbles are extremely thin and allow a gas such as air to diffuse out and go back into the solution in the blood. Optison is a perfluoropropane-filled albumin shell. Greater enhancement is observed by these agents with added advantage of low solubility.

Selective uptake agents: The colloidal suspensions of liquids such as perfluorocarbons and certain agents with durable shells are taken up by the reticuloendothelial system from where they are ultimately excreted. They may provide contrast within the liver parenchyma, demarcating the distribution of Kupffer cells. Levovist has been shown to provide late phase enhancement in the parenchyma of the liver and spleen after clearing from the vascular system.

Contrast specific imaging: Doppler detection is useful for flow in large vessels, however, does not work for flow at the parenchymal level, where the tissue is moving at the same speed or faster than the blood. Clearly a method that could identify the echo from the contrast agent and thereby suppress that from the solid tissue would provide a real time subtraction mode for contrast enhanced B mode imaging which is provided by contrast specific imaging. Unlike tissue, microbubbles scatter ultrasound in a manner depending upon their amplitude which forms the basis of clinically used contrast imaging techniques. At low incident pressures these agents produce linear backscatter enhancement. As the transmitting intensity of scanner is increased, the contrast agent begins to show nonlinear characteristics such as emission of harmonics.

This forms the basis of contrast specific imaging modes, such as harmonic, pulse inversion imaging and Doppler. As transmitting amplitude further rises contrast agents exhibit transient nonlinear scattering resulting in their destruction which forms the basis of triggered imaging. The bubbles resonate in an ultrasound field. As ultrasound wave propagates over the bubbles, the bubbles experience a periodic change in their radius in symphony with the oscillations of the incident sound. These radial oscillations have a natural or resonant frequency of oscillations at which they will both absorb and scatter ultrasound with a high efficiency. To distinguish bubbles from tissue, they are exited so as to produce harmonics and detect these in preference to the fundamental echo from the tissue.

Harmonic B mode and Doppler imaging: In harmonic mode, the system transmits normally at one frequency, but is tuned to receive echoes preferentially at double that frequency, where the echoes from the bubbles lie. Typically the transmit frequency lies between 1.5 MHz and 3 MHz and the receive frequency selected by means of a radiofrequency band pass filter, whose center frequency is at the second harmonic, between 3 MHz and 6 MHz. Echoes from solid tissues and from blood vessels are suppressed. Harmonic imaging uses the same array transducers as conventional imaging and for most of recent ultrasound systems involves only software changes. *In vivo* measurements from spectral Doppler show that the signal to noise ratio is improved by a combination of harmonic imaging and the contrast agent by as much as 35 dB. Applications of this method include detection of flow in small vessels that is moving surrounded by tissue. Low velocity detection requires lowering the Doppler PRF, which results in multiple aliasing artifacts and loss of directional resolution. Because it maps a parameter directly related to acoustic quantity that is enhanced by the contrast agent, the power Doppler is natural choice for contrast enhanced color Doppler studies. The advantage of the power map is the contrast enhanced detection of small vessel flow. Harmonic power Doppler effectively overcomes noise produced by contrast agent and is capable of demonstrating flow in very small vessels.

Pulse inversion imaging: In pulse inversion-phase imaging, two pulses are sent in rapid succession into the tissue. The second pulse is the mirror image of the first, i.e. it has undergone 180° phase change. The scanner detects the echoes from these two successive pulses and forms their sum. For ordinary tissue, which behaves in linear manner, the sum of two inverted pulses is zero. For an echo with nonlinear component such as a bubble, the echoes produced from these two pulses will not be simple mirror images of each other, because of the asymmetrical behavior of the bubble radius with time. The result is that the sum of these two echoes is not zero and a signal is detected from bubble but not from tissue. This summed echo contains the non linear and harmonic components of the signal, including the second harmonic. Pulse inversion imaging provides better suppression of linear echoes than harmonic imaging and is effective over the full bandwidth of the transducer, showing improvement of image resolution over harmonic mode. A recent development seeks to make generalization of the pulse inversion method, called pulse inversion Doppler. This technique which is also known as "power pulse inversion imaging" combines the nonlinear detection performance of pulse inversion imaging with the motion discrimination capabilities of power Doppler. Multiple transient pulses of alternating polarities are used and Doppler signal processing techniques are applied to distinguish between bubble echoes and echoes from moving tissues and/or tissue harmonics. This method offers potential improvements in the agent to tissue contrast and signal to noise performance.

Intermittent and triggered imaging: As the incident pressure to which resonating bubble is exposed is increased, the microbubble will break due to energy such intense ultrasound. As it breaks by this transient disruption, it emits a strong brief nonlinear echo. The detection of this echo forms the basis of the most sensitive method to detect microbubble contrast at the perfusion level. Ultrasound field has ability, if its peak pressure is sufficiently high, to disrupt a bubble shell, and hence destroy it. As the bubble is disrupted, it releases energy, creating a strong transient echo, which is rich in harmonics. The fact that this echo is transient in nature can be exploited for its detection. One simple method is to subtract from a disruption image, a baseline image obtained either before or immediately after insonation. Intermittent Harmonic Power Doppler for Perfusion Imaging, uses a real time, low MI, nondestructive bubble imaging mode. This can be used to survey vessels in the liver. Such images show tumor vascular morphology and reveal arterialized lesion following a bolus injection of contrast and the imaging modality of choice is pulse inversion. Following this examination, a further injection is made and after the agent is seen to enter the hepatic arterial circulation, the scanner is set to high MI and frozen for an interval between 5 and 90 seconds, allowing the agent to enter the hepatic sinusoids. The scanner is unfrozen and a "flash" or "veil" is seen as the agent is disrupted revealing the entire distribution of bubbles in the liver, including those in the parenchyma. This is a liver perfusion image. Depending on the delay, this can be timed to show the arterial, portal or post-vascular phases. The preferred mode for this method is pulse inversion, which has advantage of high resolution imaging but the disadvantage of strong tissue harmonic background, or power Doppler modes, such as harmonic power Doppler or agent detection imaging.

11

Recent Advances in Ultrasound

Shailendra Savale

Recent advances in ultrasound include:

- An increased number of transducer elements in ultrasound transducers, leading to higher lateral resolution.
- Higher center frequencies in the 10 to 15 MHz range, leading to higher lateral resolution.
- Broadband transducers and increased scanner bandwidth, resulting in higher axial resolution and allowing shifting the center frequency and frequency compounding to reduce noise.
- Increased sophistication of signal processing routines, leading to better images with lower noise and higher contrast.
- Improvements in Doppler sensitivity and power Doppler, making evaluation of the vascularity of masses relatively easy. When Doppler evaluation was first promoted in the early 1980s, continuous wave Doppler was used because of its higher sensitivity. Vessels around a breast mass were examined for high velocity flow that was thought to suggest malignancy. More recently, simply looking at the number of vessels in and around a mass with color Doppler imaging has accomplished the same purpose. The interpretation of Doppler information is still controversial, but most investigators and the ATL/FDA trial agree that increased vascularity suggests malignancy.
- The biggest single advance in recent years has been 2-dimensional scanner arrays, which provide dynamic focusing in the slice thickness plane, perpendicular to the normal scan plane. This feature dramatically improves lesion contrast close to the transducer.
- *Harmonic imaging* is a procedure in which the ultrasound machine scans images at twice the frequency transmitted. This technique potentially can suppress reverberation and other near-field noise but it may limit depth of penetration and result in loss of resolution, unless the newer broadband harmonic imaging techniques are used. Harmonic imaging has been shown to reduce the number of possible complex cysts or solid masses seen at breast sonography and

improve the examiner's confidence that a lesion is in fact truly cystic and benign. The procedure also shows potential to better define the boundaries of lesions-an important feature in distinguishing benign from malignant lesions.

- *Two-dimensional transducer arrays* can now produce three-dimensional ultrasound images. Of course, 3-D image segments may be produced using other technology, but the technique is often cumbersome. An important advantage of 3-D ultrasound is that it will allow for more rapid and reproducible scans and may solve the problem of screening ultrasound. Screening ultrasound has great potential but screening the entire breast sonographically is labor-intensive and time-consuming for both sonographer and physician. A screening test should be simple, relatively cheap, and ideally should not require a physician's presence. Screening 3-D ultrasound by a technologist or sonographer would permit the radiologist or other physician to review the 3-D data set in multiple scan planes, including the radial planes. With new technologies based on ultrasound on the verge of practical usefulness, the practice of breast ultrasound will change if sonographers and sonologists embrace the new technologies, and not avoid them. Integrating ultrasound breast imaging with new nonultrasound technologies is important, and so is programs to train and accredit as many individuals and practices as possible.
- *The 4 D ultrasound* implies the real time imaging of 3D ultrasound.
- *Ultrasound contrast* agents usually employ encapsulated bubbles or solid particles in the 5 to 7-micron range, producing a marked increase in backscatter and making it easy to visualize flowing blood. They also produce moderate tissue enhancement usable for dynamic perfusion studies that look for changes in tissue enhancement over time. When some agents are exposed to a higher power ultrasound beam, the microbubbles break, releasing acoustic energy that can be detected using color or power Doppler. This phenomenon

has been called stimulated acoustic emission and may be useful for detecting contrast agents in tissue when the gray-scale imaging does not clearly show the agent. The disadvantages of contrast agents are their cost and the requirement for an intravenous injection. Also, with more sensitive Doppler instrumentation, blood flow enhancement may not be as important as it has been in the past.

- *Elastography* calculates strain produced by the tissue and characterizes stiffness of underlying tissue. Benign and malignant lesions have different stiffness. Strain imaging display relative stiffness of lesion compared to surrounding normal tissue. Stiffer areas deform less easily than surrounding. Stiffer areas appear dark and softer areas appear light. Transducer is moved over the affected area. Machine records two images simultaneously a B mode picture and an Elastogram. Both images are displayed side by side. Area on B mode and elastogram is compared. If area of stiffness is larger than B mode and appears dark with large contrast, the lesion is malignant while if area is smaller than B mode, the lesion is benign. Different scores are available to specify elasticity of lesion; the most commonly accepted is Tsukuba Elasticity Score. The score ranges from 0 to 5, more the score greater the stiffness. The zero score is given to lesion appearing green on elastography while score 5 is given for the lesion appearing blue. The score 5 is indicative of malignancy. The elastography is applied in evaluation of breast lesions, lymph nodes, thyroid lesions, skin lesions, prostatic malignancy and evaluation of liver fibrosis. Recently it is also used in evaluation of tendon injuries.

- *Endoscopic ultrasound* was introduced by Dr Charles Lightgale in 1980 for early diagnosis and precise staging of malignancy. The basic principle is to reduce the distance between ultrasound source and organ to be imaged. The target is achieved by placing ultrasound transducer at the tip of endoscope which is advanced till the target organ is visualized through the transducer. The high frequency transducer gives better resolution. The procedure includes pharyngeal anesthesia and intravenous sedation. Under direct vision, the echoendoscope is passed to the target area, and intraluminal gas is aspirated.

Image interpretation requires a thorough knowledge of anatomic relationships of intra-abdominal vessels and organs, an understanding of the general principles of ultrasound imaging. In the esophagus, the scope is usually parallel to the wall so that the sonographic plane and the wall are perpendicular to each other for optimal imaging.

It is extremely accurate in staging non-Hodgkins lymphoma of the gastrointestinal tract. The benign lymph nodes appear triangular while malignant appear oval in shape. It has a great role in monitoring the progression of the disease during chemotherapy and demonstrating complete disappearance of the intramural infiltration and reappearance of the normal five-layer wall architecture. In imaging carcinoma esophagus, the relationship of the lesion to extra-esophageal mediastinal structures, such as the aorta, trachea, and heart can be made. It gives more appropriate staging of the carcinoma. In gastric carcinoma, except for tumors that do not break through the mucosal surface, such as linitis plastica, conventional endoscopy is superior to endoscopic ultrasound for diagnosis. It is superior to other modalities in visualization of pancreatic lesion less than 2 cm. For bigger lesion CT, ultrasound, ERCP are equally effective. A short optimal focal range of only 4 cm and difficulty in differentiation of focal chronic pancreatitis from carcinoma are the limiting factors. It is the most accurate method of clinically staging neoplastic disorders of the gastrointestinal tract. It is not only essential for staging, but can also provide unique diagnostic information, often otherwise obtainable only by laparotomy or resection.

- *High-intensity Focused Ultrasound (HIFU)*

The use of ultrasound in clinical practice is no longer limited to diagnostic imaging or to simple needle guidance in the performance of percutaneous procedures such as amniocentesis or tumor biopsy. Ultrasound technology now allows the use of focused ultrasound energy for therapeutic purposes such as tissue ablation and hemostasis. High-intensity focused ultrasound is being promoted as a noninvasive method to treat certain primary solid tumors and metastatic disease, to ablate foci of ectopic electrical activity in the heart, and to achieve hemostasis in acute traumatic injuries to the extremities and visceral organs. The field of medicine is evolving toward greater use of noninvasive and minimally invasive therapies such as HIFU. Unlike radiofrequency or cryoablation, which are also used to ablate tumors, ultrasound is completely noninvasive and can be used to reach areas of hemorrhage or tumors that are deep within the body, provided there is an acoustic window to allow the transmission of ultrasound energy. Preliminary reports suggest that there is reduced toxicity with HIFU ablation compared with other ablation techniques because of the noninvasive nature of the procedure. As early as 1954, Lindstrom and Fry investigated the possibility of using high-intensity ultrasound for treating neurologic disorders in humans. Fry and colleagues are credited with the first application of HIFU in humans by producing elevated acoustic intensities *in vivo* by focusing ultrasound energy in a manner analogous to the way a magnifying glass can be used to focus light. In comparing the differences in intensities of HIFU and diagnostic ultrasound, HIFU has significantly higher time-averaged intensities in the focal region of the ultrasound transducer. Typical diagnostic ultrasound transducers deliver ultrasound with time-averaged intensities of approximately 0.1 to 100 mW/cm^2 or compression and rarefaction pressures of 0.001 to 0.003 MPa, depending on the mode of imaging (B-mode, pulsed Doppler sonography, or continuous wave Doppler sonography). In contrast, HIFU transducers deliver ultrasound with intensities in the range of 100 to 10,000 W/cm^2 to the focal region, with peak compression pressures of up to 30 MPa and peak rarefaction pressures up to 10 MPa. The major effect of high acoustic intensities in tissue is heat generation due to absorption of the acoustic energy. The heat raises the temperature rapidly to 60°C or higher in the tissue, causing coagulation necrosis within a few seconds. Focusing results in high intensities at a specific location and over only a small volume (e.g. 1 mm diameter and 9 mm length). This focusing minimizes the potential for thermal damage to tissue located between the transducer and the focal point because the intensities are much lower outside the focal region. Mechanical phenomena, in addition to thermal effects, are associated at high intensities but are not present at lower intensities. Mechanical phenomena include cavitation, microstreaming, and radiation forces. Cavitation can be defined as the creation or motion of a gas cavity in an acoustic field; for example, the oscillatory movement of a gas-filled bubble in a liquid medium exposed to an acoustic field. Cavitation occurs due to alternating compression and expansion of tissue as an ultrasound field propagates through it. If the tissue expansion or rarefaction pressure is of sufficient magnitude, gas can be extracted from the tissue, resulting in bubble formation. This bubble can then further interact with the ultrasound field. There are two forms of cavitation to consider. The first is stable cavitation, in which a bubble is exposed to a low-pressure acoustic field, resulting in stable oscillation of the size of the bubble. The other is inertial cavitation, in which the exposure of the bubble to the acoustic field results in violent oscillations of the bubble and rapid growth of the bubble during the rarefaction phase, eventually leading to the violent collapse and destruction of the bubble. An interesting phenomenon has been observed when inertial cavitation occurs against a solid surface. The asymmetric collapse of a bubble near such a surface can create high-velocity liquid jets

that impinge on the surface with a force sufficient to damage metal surfaces and disrupt cell membranes. If inertial cavitation occurs near a cell membrane, one may anticipate mechanical, rather than thermal, damage to the cell. Stable cavitation may lead to a phenomenon called "microstreaming" (rapid movement of fluid near the bubble due to its oscillating motion). Microstreaming can produce high shear forces close to the bubble that can disrupt cell membranes and may play a role in ultrasound-enhanced drug or gene delivery when damage to the cell membrane is transient. Radiation forces are developed when a wave is either absorbed or reflected. Complete reflection produces twice the force that complete absorption does. These forces are constant if the amplitude of a wave is steady and the absorption or reflection is constant. If the reflecting or absorbing medium is tissue or other solid material, the force presses against the medium, producing a pressure termed "radiation pressure." If the medium is liquid and can move under pressure, then streaming results. Diagnostic ultrasound has an excellent safety profile, with no clinically significant deleterious biologic effects having been reported using current diagnostic equipment. However, at high intensities, ultrasound can result in tissue heating and necrosis, cell apoptosis, and cell lysis. Mechanisms involved in HIFU-induced biologic effects are primarily caused by thermal and cavitation mechanisms, as discussed previously. Coagulation necrosis occurs in tissue exposed to high-intensity ultrasound when the temperature of the tissue is elevated to a certain level for a certain time. The temperature required to induce coagulation necrosis is time-dependent. Tissue temperature elevated to more than 60°C for 1 second will generally lead to instantaneous cell death via coagulation necrosis in most tissues, which is the primary mechanism for tumor cell destruction in HIFU therapy. Although most initial cell death in tissues exposed to HIFU fields is caused by cell necrosis from thermal injury, HIFU can also induce apoptosis. In apoptotic cells, the nucleus of the cell self-destructs with rapid degradation of DNA by endonucleases. The primary mechanism of cell death by hyperthermia is apoptosis. Apoptosis has also been shown in leukemic cells exposed to low-intensity ultrasound and in leukemic cells exposed to ultrasound-induced cavitation. Apoptosis may be an important delayed bioeffect in tissue exposed to low-energy HIFU, especially in cell types that regenerate poorly, such as neurons. Hence, there may be a more extensive area of cellular death than just the target area of the HIFU, and this mechanism might be a potential limitation of the technique because cell death due to apoptosis occurs at a lower level of energy deposition than occurs during

HIFU, and tissue adjacent to the target may be at risk from this effect. Finally, nonlinear effects are observed at high acoustic intensities. As a high-intensity acoustic wave propagates through water or tissue, the wave can become distorted so that a sinusoidal wave initially generated by an ultrasound transducer can become sawtooth-shaped due to conversion of energy carried in the fundamental frequency to higher harmonics, which are more rapidly absorbed. This process results in more rapid attenuation of the ultrasound energy and more rapid tissue heating. This can also have the effect of distorting the distribution of heat production that would be predicted if nonlinear effects did not occur. A better understanding of nonlinear effects in biologic systems will be critical for advancing clinical HIFU. To date, the contribution of each of these effects remains poorly understood. Tissue specimens obtained after HIFU ablation of prostate gland, for example, show incomplete destruction of tissue by coagulation necrosis; and to our knowledge no follow-up studies exist at this time to determine the ultimate extent of tissue destruction by apoptosis. Dose delivery to targeted tissues depends on the transducer array, the energy input, and the tissue attenuation that occurs between the transducer and the target. With more research, it may be possible to control which type of effect is being induced in the targeted tissues, but for now the ablative effect of HIFU is a combination of all of them.

LIMITATIONS OF HIFU

Although it offers tremendous potential for noninvasive therapy of malignancies, particularly those that are widespread or inoperable, the usefulness of HIFU has limitations, and risk is associated with its use that could result in adverse outcomes. Because HIFU is essentially ultrasound, any artifacts related to ultrasound would apply to HIFU as well, such as acoustic shadowing, reverberation, and refraction. Hence, lesions that are deep in relation to bones, such as a liver lesion adjacent to a rib, will be difficult to treat. Gas in bowel cannot be penetrated by HIFU just as it cannot be with diagnostic sonography. These sound waves are reflected back toward the transducer. With diagnostic sonography, these reflected sound waves are of such low energy that there is no adverse effect from them. However, with HIFU, these reflected waves are very high energy, and they can produce burns in the tissues that lie between the transducer and the target. In our experience, even small amounts of gas in the gastrointestinal tract can produce burns in the wall of the bowel anterior to the gas and in the abdominal wall musculature overlying the gas. Refraction artifacts can result in energy deposition in the soft tissues adjacent to the target area, and energy deposition can occur superficially to the target if the ultrasound beam is not carefully focused into a small point. The amount of energy absorbed by the tissues is essentially estimated by making the assumption that the attenuation of the sound waves in the soft tissues between the transducer and the target is linear. This assumption may not always be true; and fibrotic, fatty, and highly vascularized tissues attenuate sound energy differently. Excessive energy absorption can lead to unpredictable distributions of cell death. Hence, targeting is of extreme importance, which is why magnetic resonance (MR) guidance for HIFU has initially become more rapidly accepted clinically than sonographically guided HIFU. One potential complication of HIFU is the dissemination of malignant cells from the shear forces generated by the procedure, but this potential complication has not been substantiated either *in vitro* or *in vivo*. Great care will be necessary in treating patients with HIFU to ensure that complications do not occur.

IMAGING GUIDANCE AND MONITORING OF THERAPY

Guidance and monitoring of acoustic therapy is most important to ensure that the desired region is treated and to minimize damage to adjacent structures. Monitoring using real-time imaging, such as with sonography, ensures that the targeting of the HIFU beam is maintained on the correct area throughout the procedure. Currently, MR and sonography are being used for guidance and monitoring of HIFU therapy. Both methods have their advantages and disadvantages. MR has the advantage of providing temperature data within seconds after HIFU exposure. However, MR guidance is expensive, labor-intensive, and of lower spatial resolution in some cases, although it is superior to sonography in obese patients. Sonographic guidance provides the benefit of imaging using the same form of energy that is being used for therapy. The significance of this is that the acoustic window can be verified with sonography. Therefore, if the target cannot be well visualized with sonography, then it is unlikely that HIFU therapy will be effective in the target region, and it may potentially cause thermal injury to unintended tissue. Temperature monitoring using sonography is not yet available, although sonographic thermometry is being actively investigated and a clinical HIFU device in China has an incorporated sonographic thermometry system. In some instances when tissue contrast is not sufficient to visualize a tumor in the background of normal tissue, elastography may prove helpful. Imaging methods to assess HIFU treatment are similar to those used to assess the response to other methods of ablation such as radiofrequency ablation and include contrast enhanced CT and MR. In addition, the use of microbubble contrast-enhanced sonography is also being examined as a method to evaluate the treatment effect of HIFU. These methods all examine the change in vascularity of the treated volume. Another method currently being examined in oncologic applications is the use of PET to assess for changes in metabolic activity after HIFU treatment.

CURRENT CLINICAL APPLICATIONS

The investigation and applications of HIFU are growing rapidly. The major application of HIFU clinically is for the treatment of benign and malignant solid tumors. Several other potential therapeutic applications of HIFU are being investigated, including thrombolysis, arterial occlusion for the treatment of tumors and bleeding, hemostasis of bleeding vessels and organs, and drug and gene delivery. To date, studies using animals and human subjects have been published for the treatment of hepatocellular carcinoma (HCC), renal cell carcinoma, pancreatic cancer, some sarcomas, urinary bladder tumors, and prostate carcinoma. HCC is rapidly becoming the most common malignancy worldwide. Surgery, particularly liver transplantation, offers the only real hope for cure; survival rates are only 25-30% at 5 years. As a result, noninvasive alternatives to surgery, such as radiofrequency ablation, ethanol injection, and HIFU, have generated increasing interest as alternative or adjunct treatments to surgery. Animal models for the assessment of HIFU devices have been published. Small-animal models have established that HIFU can ablate areas of normal liver, and energy thresholds for liver tissue destruction have been published. Further small-animal experiments have correlated the histology of HIFU with tissue depth intensity levels. Pig liver specimens have been used to show that the site for ablation can be accurately placed.

HIGH INTENSITY FOCUSED ULTRASOUND TECHNOLOGY

To deposit large amounts of energy deep into the body without causing damage to tissue in the prefocal or postfocal region, it is necessary to use a wide aperture system that delivers acoustic energy with a beam that has a large angle of convergence. Some units have been produced with an aperture as large as 40 cm. Critical to the performance of HIFU, just as with diagnostic imaging, is the ability to obtain an adequate acoustic window to allow propagation of acoustic energy to the target. An acoustic window is an area through which a sonogram of the structures within can be obtained. There are a limited number of such acoustic windows because bone, air, and gas interfere with the propagation of ultrasound beams into the body, thus obscuring targets beyond these interfaces. For example, the bladder is an excellent acoustic window, and treatment results of urinary bladder tumors with HIFU have been published. Three-dimensional sonography may provide information that would be valuable to the performance of HIFU. Three-dimensional sonography is likely to better delineate a volume of tissue to be treated than just a single plane or orthogonal planes, and most commercially available HIFU systems display with 2D sonography systems. Therefore, the application of 3D sonography techniques is an exciting area of future opportunity, especially for HIFU treatment planning and monitoring. HIFU has the potential to allow completely noninvasive treatment of tumors. The main advantage of HIFU is its ability to deposit high amounts of energy deep inside the body and tissue, with millimeter accuracy and little or no damage to intervening tissue. In some applications, no sedation or anesthesia is used during the delivery of HIFU therapy. HIFU is being increasingly used for limited applications in Asia and Europe; however, these studies have all been preliminary, and further investigation will be necessary before the widespread use of HIFU can be recommended. With advances in imaging and transducer technology and better understanding of HIFU-related bioeffects, HIFU is likely to gain acceptance clinically as a technique for noninvasive ablation of tissue for oncologic applications.

INTRAVASCULAR ULTRASOUND

It is defined as acquisition of cross-sectional images of the target vessel by an ultrasound probe placed on the tip of an endoluminally positioned catheter.

The advantages of intravascular ultrasound are, full circumference of vessel wall can be visualized, and electronically generated scale that negates the need for radiographic magnification, qualitative information, response to interventional strategies can be evaluated.

The intravascular ultrasound can be done by five methods, conventional gray-scale intravascular ultrasound (IVUS), color flow IVUS, virtual histology mapping, integrated backscatter IVUS and microbubbles.

Conventional Gray Scale IVUS

In conventional gray-scale IVUS intensity of reflected signals collected by the IVUS transducer enables creation of conventional grey-scale images. Elastin and collagen organization within vessel wall provides different scattering properties between the individual layers.

Equipment

Catheter with miniature transducer at its tip, 2 types of catheter systems are end-hole catheter delivered over guidewire and catheters delivered directly through the sheath. Two main transducer designs are phased-array and mechanical type. The console for image reconstruction uses frequency centred at 12.5–20 MHz, upto 40 MHz. The main two types of transducers can be used. The main differences are given in Table 11.1.

Normal Arterial Anatomy on IVUS

Blood is seen as characteristic speckled pattern, constantly changing in echogenicity with cardiac cycle, slightly more echogenic in systole. When blood flow is slow and stagnant, increased backscatter may give false impression of thrombus/plaque. Intima appears as thin echogenic layer and requires high frequency for proper resolution. The internal elastic lamina appears as thin highly echogenic layer. Blooming may cause overestimation of actual thickness, making it difficult to distinguish from mild intimal proliferation. In the media echogenicity depends on relative content of smooth muscle, collagen and elastin. Elastic arteries have a strongly echo reflective media, less marked distinction and layered/homogeneous appearance. The adventitia is collagen-rich outermost bright layer.

In atherosclerosis it determines plaque composition (Table 11.2) rather than stenotic severity that determines vulnerability of a lesion to rupture. The Table 11.2 gives the appearance of the plaque that indicates the content of the plaque.

The thrombus appears echogenic, typical scintillating or sparkling pattern on ultrasound with presence of microchannels and echodensity of less than 50% of that of adventitia.

IVUS can detect the presence of hypoechoic media to distinguish a true from a false aneurysm, even when the media is greatly thinned out. Mistaking a false lumen for true lumen can have serious consequences if the former is selected for stent or graft placements.

IVUS helps by recognition of characteristic 3-layered appearance of true lumen, side branches arising from true lumen and slow flowing, more echogenic blood within false lumen.

Limitations of Conventional IVUS

Sensitivity of imaging is affected by, frequency of transducer, gain settings, depth of penetration, focal depth and lipid content, Location and orientation of imaging probe within the arterial lumen influences the vessel wall structure. Lateral impulse response artifacts occur when catheter is eccentrically placed,

Table 11.1 Difference between phased array and mechanical transducer

Phased-array transducer	Mechanical transducer
1. Coupled with smaller catheters	1. Require relatively larger catheters
2. Flexible, guided into small tortuous vessels easily	2. Stiffer, traversing aortic bifurcation or reaching visceral vessels difficult
3. No such problem	3. Nonuniform rotation maybe a problem due to a drive cable and moving parts
4. Easily incorporated into interventional devices	4. Difficult to do so
5. Complex design	5. Simple design
6. Expensive	6. Less costly

Table 11.2 The composition of the plaque with its ultrasound charactristics

Appearance	Content
Hypoechoic	High lipid content
Soft echoes	Fibromuscular tissue
Hyperechoic	Collagen rich fibrous plaque
Hyperechoic with distal shadowing	Plaque calcification

i.e. false positive intimal flap or ulceration, Dark images obtained make distinction of lumen from echolucent plaque, neointimal hyperplasia, and mural thrombus difficult. The distinction of atherosclerotic plaque from underlying media is also difficult. Lesions at intimal surface may sometimes not be adequately visualized because they fall below the resolution limit of the IVUS system or they are obscured by contents of atherosclerotic plaque. Deep calcifications within the atherosclerotic plaque may limit the ability to correctly evaluate the diameter of stenosis. Imaging of intracranial circulation has been limited due to narrow course and marked tortuosity of the vessels, making navigation difficult.

Color Flow IVUS

Real-time images are produced from the transducer at 30 frames/sec and difference between 2 adjacent frames is detected by computer software producing the colored images. The red denotes movement of echogenic blood particles through artery. The red to orange implies vascular stenosis resulting in increased velocity of blood.

Advantages of color flow IVUS are, distinction of luminal blood flow from dark echolucent plaque along along vessel wall, accurate stent deployment due to greater understanding of lumen size and blood flow, no need of conventional angiography in patients with renal failure or contrast allergy, study of blood flow following interventional procedures and high image resolution.

Limitations of Color Flow IVUS includes short scanning diameter, entire lumen may not generate colored intensity, especially if probe is directed against the vessel wall, or if large caliber sheaths are used, flow velocity cannot be calculated, it cannot be performed along with virtual histology imaging and it is not gated with heart rate.

Virtual Histology Mapping

Various components of vessel wall reflect signal intensity differently, creating an opportunity for histological details to be detected and mapped with color coding. With auto-regressive analysis of signals, real-time dynamic assessment can be done The following table gives color codes for the virtual histology mapping (Table 11.3).

Limitations of virtual histology mapping includes, interpretation of results requires experience, it cannot be used simultaneously with color flow, it is time consuming process, metal stents maybe misread as calcifications and overestimation of necrotic core of plaque.

Integrated Backscatter IVUS

It is a technique of producing a color coded map of the atherosclerotic plaque (Table 11.4) which reflects the tissue characteristics of plaque composition using a different algorithm than virtual histology mapping.

The following table gives color codes for composition of plaque.

Advantages

This is accurate tissue characteristics in quantity and quality than virtual histology mapping technique.

Table 11.3 Color codes in virtual histology mapping

Dark green	Fibrous material
Yellow/green	Fibrofatty content
White	Calcified deposit
Red	Necrotic lipid core

Table 11.4 Color codes for composition of plaque in Integrated Backscatter IVUS

Green	Fibrous tissue
Yellow	Dense fibrosis
Blue	Lipid pool
Red	Calcification

Limitations

Tissue characterization is distorted when lesions are not perpendicular to the probe. Also angle of dependence required for accurate visualization depends on strength of signal of IVUS equipment; plaques largely composed of calcified or fibrous tissue have a larger angular scattering behavior versus normal or fatty plaque, heavy calcification obscures the view of deeper tissues, acoustic shadowing by metal stents hinders the viewing of deeper tissues and it can be time consuming and requires reader expertise.

Microbubbles

Site-targeted acoustic contrast agents are being developed to further identify specific vascular pathology as an adjunct to IVUS by accurately enhancing intraluminal contours. Most studies have focussed on coronary circulation, with very limited study of the carotid circulation.

Proliferation of vasa vasorum and intraplaque hemorrhage precedes or occurs concomitantly with plaque inflammation and instability. Increased neovascularization of vasa vasorum and plaques can be traced with contrast-enhanced IVUS. Lipid microbubbles are used to identify intra-plaque inflammation because these lipid microbubbles are phagocytosed by macrophages within the inflamed plaque. Subsequently the phagocytosed microbubbles generate characteristic echogenic features that can be used to identify their distribution within the plaque with real-time IVUS.

Clinical Applications of IVUS

- Identification of arterial plaques in high-risk asymptomatic patients, so that timely treatment can be rendered.
- By differentiating a stenosis produced by thrombus, plaque or mural abnormality, IVUS helps to select appropriate recanalization technique.
- Stenoses is better visualized and characterized on the basis of composition, plaque area and percentage stenosis which may guide the choice of treatment.
- It helps in accurate determination of balloon size.
- It helps in accurate degree of apposition of stent to vessel wall.
- It helps in determination of exact location and depth of plaque for atherectomy. IVUS can also identify superficial calcification which is associated with poor tissue retrieval. Evaluation of post-procedural residual plaque burden can be imaged.
- It helps in accurate determination of diameter of proximal and distal neck of aneurysm to

select correct size of stent graft for endovascular treatment of aneurysms.

- IVUS can be used to complement cavography in case of technical problems, e.g. filter tilting or migration, or complications, e.g. Caval thrombosis or recurrent pulmonary embolism. Also, identification of renal veins is easy with IVUS.
- In case of aortic dissection, IVUS is superior to angiography and transesophageal echo-cardiography in identifying points of entry and re-entry. Percutaneous fenestration of aortic dissection has been accomplished successfully using IVUS as guiding modality. Identification of highly echogenic needle as it passes from one lumen to another is easily monitored by IVUS.
- Mechanisms of restenosis following angioplasty, with emphasis to positive and negative remodelling of vessel wall, have been adequately studied by means of IVUS.
- To study the effect of pharmacological and non-pharmacological interventions on progression or stabilization of atherosclerosis.
- Diagnosis and follow-up of patients with Marfan's syndrome (abnormalities of elastin content).

Relatively safe procedure. It is difficult to maneuver the catheter through heavily stenotic or tortuous vessels. Catheter may disrupt an atherosclerotic plaque in areas of high grade stenosis leading to embolic phenomena. Heparinization during procedure may be helpful. Rare cases of arterial dissection and perforation have been reported.

Limitations of IVUS

It may be difficult to differentiate thrombus superimposed upon plaque from a soft lipid laden plaque, it may be unable to maintain a constant catheter-vessel coaxial alignment, calcific/fibrous lesions may cause echo dropouts, hindering the vision of underlying plaque, high cost of equipment, increased time of procedure, it requires operator expertise and due to lack of standardization IVUS catheters cannot be exchanged between different manufacturers.

FUTURE UTILITY

Continued improvements in transducer design will allow better resolution and penetration of ultrasound waves, improvements in catheter trackability and steerability will allow easier catheterization of tortuous vessels and side branches, incorporation of IVUS as part of the interventional radiologist's armamentarium will positively impact operator's decision during therapeutic procedures and will help evaluate impact of this modality on long-term outcomes and it may ultimately decrease postprocedural complication rates.

12

Mammography

Hariqbal Singh

Mammography requires consistent high-quality images with optimum film density, contrast, high resolution and low radiation dose. It is particularly important in diagnosing small cancers as they may be subtle. The mammography equipment and technique used therefore have to take into account wide variation in breast size, variation in the relative amounts of fat, glandular and stromal tissue which are present, and the low contrast between normal breast tissue and common pathological lesions.

Technical principles for dedicated mammography X-ray equipment to produce high-quality images include.

- *Generator:* Most modern high-voltage generators produce a near constant potential output using medium- or high-frequency converter technology. A high output rate is desirable in order to reduce exposure time and therefore minimize movement unsharpness.

- *X-ray tube:* The most commonly used target-filter combination is a molybdenum (Mo) target with 0.03 mm Mo filter. The peak kilovoltage is normally in the range 26 to 30 kV and typically 28 kV. The resultant X-ray spectrum exhibits characteristic X-rays at 17.4 and 19.4 keV, with a sharp cut-off above 20 keV due to the absorption edge for molybdenum. The remaining lower energy photons, mainly in the range 17 to 20 keV, are well suited for producing maximum contrast from the radiographically similar soft tissues of the breast. The Mo/Mo target filter combination is well suited for the average or small sized breast. Large breasts or breasts containing high proportion of glandular tissue may require a higher energy spectrum of energy radiation to provide sufficient penetration. Therefore certain mammography machines have a choice of target—filter combinations including Mo/Mo, Mo/rhodium, Mo/palladium and rhodium/rhodium. As small focal spot is necessary for high resolution images. A focal spot size of 0.3 to 0.35 mm is used in normal mammography. A fine focal spot of 0.1 mm is used in magnification

mammography. The focus to film distance varies from 60 to 65 cm.

- *Automatic exposure controller:* The AEC automatically controls the exposure duration so that the optimum optical density of the mammograms is maintained over a wide range of different breast sizes and densities. The AEC device, either a photo-timer or ionization chamber, is normally positioned 3 to 5 cm posterior to the nipple, where the densest glandular tissue is likely to be situated.

- *Secondary radiation grid:* The use of a moving grid system results in improved resolution and contrast by decreasing scattered radiation. The potential increase in dose due to use of a grid can be offset by use of faster film-screen combinations. A grid is not necessary for magnification mammography where the scattered radiation is removed by the air gap.

- *Compression:* Firm compression is essential for high-quality mammograms and is applied using a powered system operated by a foot control. It is important that there is even compression of the entire breast. The effects of compression are: (i) Reduced dose; (ii) Reduced scatter-improved contrast; (iii) Reduced geometric unsharpness; (iv) Reduced movement unsharpness; (v) Reduced range of breast thickness; (vi) Reduced tissue overlap improved resolution.

- *Film-screen combination:* Single side emulsion film is used with a single intensifying screen in order to ensure optimum resolution. Specially designed cassettes ensure good film-screen contact and have a front face constructed of low radiation absorption material. Modern screens use rare earth materials, e.g. gadolinium oxysulfide, which increase the speed of the film-screen combination, allowing a decrease in the radiation dose required while maximizing contrast.

- *Processing:* Dedicated processing facilities should be available for mammography film to obtain consistently highest quality images. The chosen processing conditions and chemistry need to be matched to the film-screen combination in use. In general, optimum film density and contrast are achieved by an extended processing time of up to 3.5 minutes together with a lower developer temperature (34°C) than for general radiography.

The American College of Radiologists set up standards for rating mammograms, which is called breast imaging reporting and data system (BIRADS).

BREAST IMAGING REPORTING AND DATA SYSTEM CLASSIFICATIONS

BI-RADS 0: Need additional imaging evaluation and/or prior mammograms for comparison.

BI-RADS 0 are utilized when further imaging evaluation by means of additional views or ultrasound or by retrieval of prior films is required.

BI-RADS 1 is a negative thereby meaning that the breasts are normal. The breasts are symmetric and no masses, architectural distortion or suspicious calcifications.

BI-RADS 2 is used to describe a benign finding like fibroadenoma, multiple secretory calcifications, and fat-containing lesions such as oil cysts, lipomas, galactoceles and mixed-density hamartomas in the mammography report with no mammographic evidence of malignancy.

BI-RADS 3 is probably benign finding. A finding placed in this category should have less than a 2% risk of malignancy. Lesions appropriately placed in this category include nonpalpable, circumscribed mass on a baseline mammogram, focal asymmetry which becomes less dense on spot compression view or a cluster of punctate calcifications. The initial short-term follow-up is a unilateral mammogram at 6 months, then a bilateral follow-up examination at 12 months and 24 months after the initial examination. If the findings show no change in the follow-up the final assessment is changed to BI-RADS 2 (benign) and no further follow-up is required. If a BI-RADS 3 lesion shows any change during follow-up, it will change into a BI-RADS 4 or 5 and appropriate action should be taken.

BI-RADS 4 is a suspicious abnormality. This category is reserved for findings that do not have the classic appearance of malignancy but have a wide range of probability of malignancy in 2 to 95% of cases. Biopsy should be considered.

BI-RADS 5 is highly suggestive of malignancy. It must be reserved for findings that are classic of breast cancers, with >95% likelihood of malignancy. A spiculated, irregular high-density mass, a segmental or linear arrangement of fine linear calcifications or an irregular spiculated mass with associated pleomorphic calcifications are lesions placed in BI-RADS 5.

BI-RADS 6 is a known biopsy proven malignancy. It is reserved for lesions identified on the imaging study with biopsy confirmation of malignancy prior to definitive therapy.

13

Computed Tomography

Varsha Rangankar

Computed tomography (CT) is the science that creates two-dimensional cross sectional images from three-dimensional body structures. "Tomos" is the Greek word for "cut" or "section", and tomography is a technique for digitally cutting a specimen open using X-rays to reveal its interior details. A CT image is typically called a slice, as it corresponds to a slice from a loaf of bread. This analogy is fitting, because just as a slice of bread has a thickness, a CT slice corresponds to a certain thickness of the object being scanned. Therefore, whereas a typical digital image is composed of pixels (picture elements), a CT slice image is composed of voxels (volume elements). CT was invented in 1972 by two scientists Godfrey Hounsfield from Great Britain and Allan Cormack from United States which earned them the Nobel Prize for medicine in 1979. The first CT scanner, an EMI Mark 1 produced images with 80×80 pixel resolutions (3 mm pixels) and each slice required approximately 4.5 minutes of scanning time and 1.5 minutes of reconstruction time.

Computed Tomography (CT) is a very advanced and complicated form of X-ray imaging and provides the most diagnostic information of any ionizing radiation imaging system. An X-ray tube is used to take thousands of individual X-ray images that are digitized and processed by a computer to create very accurate cross sectional images. These cross section images provide differentiation between various types of soft tissue including gray matter, white matter, blood, tumor, muscle, fat, etc. In its most basic form, fundamental principle of CT is same as that of radiography with respect that X-rays are directed through an object to recreate an image of original object based on X-ray absorption of object. Tomography is a process that uses the movement of the X-ray tube and X-ray detector to focus the image at a specific depth or plane inside the object being imaged. The X-ray tube and detector are moved together about a fulcrum located at the level of the focal plane. Any structures inside the object that are not on the focal plane become blurred by the movement of the X–ray beam. Tomography allows the radiographer to capture a single, one film, image of a thin layer inside the patient's body. In CT imaging a computer is used to calculate and construct a digital tomographic image from thousands of images taken as the X-ray head travels in an arc around the patient and therefore the traditional tomographic blurring effect is not used in CT imaging. Each view or individual X-ray image keeps all the body structures in focus. Thus CT is display of anatomy of thin slices of body developed from multiple X-ray absorption (attenuation) measurement made around body's periphery. A mathematical back projection algorithm combines these individual views or images into a single cross-sectional image, looking $90°$ to X-ray beam (transverse section). Further digital image processing combines multiple transverse section images to create sagittal and coronal views.

Fundamentally, a CT scanner makes many measurements of attenuation through the plane of a finite-thickness cross section of the body. The system uses these data to reconstruct a digital image of the cross section, with each pixel in the image representing a measurement of the mean attenuation of a boxlike element (voxel) that extends through the thickness of the section. An attenuation measurement quantifies the fraction of radiation removed in passing through a given amount of a specific material of thickness x. Attenuation is expressed as follows:

Where,

I = X-ray intensity measured with the material in the X-ray beam path,

I_0 = X-ray intensity measured without the material in the X-ray beam path, and

m = linear attenuation coefficient of the specific material.

Basic equation - $I = I_0 e^{-mx}$

I_0 = incident intensity

I = transmitted intensity

e = Euler's constant (2.718)

m = linear attenuation coefficient

x = thickness of object

The gray levels in a CT slice correspond to X-ray attenuation, which reflects the proportion of X-rays scattered or absorbed as they pass through each voxel. Attenuation depends on atomic number and density of material through which X-ray pass and energy spectrum of incident X-rays. The internal structure of an object is reconstructed from multiple projections of object and attenuation measurements are added to produce numeric representation of an object. Although numeric representation contain all the information of process, it is difficult to interpret thus this is converted to picture form by assigning gray scale to numbers. CT is the technology that was made possible by the invention of computer. As mentioned CT is a mathematical process and utilizes a mathematical technique called reconstruction to accomplish this task. In a basic sense, a CT image is the result of breaking apart a three-dimensional structure and mathematically putting it back together again and displaying it as a two-dimensional image on a television screen. Modern computers deliver the computational power that allows the reconstruction of the image data virtually in real time. The primary goal of any CT system is to accurately reproduce the internal structures of the body as two-dimensional cross-sectional images. This goal is accomplished by computed tomography's superior ability to overcome superimposition of structures and demonstrate slight differences in tissue contrast. The collection of many projections of an object and heavy filtration of the X-ray beam play important roles in CT image formation. Each component of a CT system plays a major role in the accurate formation of each CT image. All CT systems use three step process to generate CT image that are scanning and data acquisition, reconstruction and display.

Various definitions used are following as:

- Voxel = small attenuating volume of material.
- Ray projection/ray sums= single attenuation measurement.
- Matrix-display of CT numbers in grid of squares manner
- Pixel-single square of matrix
- Window width-selecting number of gray shades for image display
- Window level—the number at which window is centered.

SYSTEM CONFIGURATION

CT gantry: The first major component of a CT system is referred to as the scan or imaging system. The imaging system primarily includes the gantry and patient table or couch. The gantry is a moveable structural frame that contains the X-ray tube including collimators and filters, detectors, data acquisition system (DAS), rotational components including slip ring systems and all associated electronics such as gantry angulation motors and positioning laser lights. It has central aperture within which patient lies. A CT gantry can be angled up to 30° toward a forward or backward position allowing the operator to align pertinent anatomy with the scanning plane. Gantry angulation is determined by the manufacturer and varies among CT systems. The opening through which a patient passes is referred to as the gantry aperture with diameters ranging from 50 to 85 cm. The larger gantry aperture allows for easier manipulation of biopsy equipment and reduces the risk of injury when scanning the patient and the placement of the biopsy needle simultaneously. The diameter of the gantry aperture is different for the diameter of the scanning circle or scan field of view. Generally, the scanning diameter in which patient or projection data is acquired is less than the size of the gantry aperture. Lasers or high intensity lights are included within or mounted on the gantry, serving as anatomical positioning guides that reference the center of the axial, coronal, and sagittal planes.

X-ray generators: Most CT scanners today use high frequency generators to produce X-ray quanta required for today's modern CT protocols. The typical operating frequency range from 5 to 50 kHz and Generator power can range from 15 to 60 KW which support exposure technique from 80 to 140 kV and 30 to 500 mA. In older CT systems a small generator supplied power to the X-ray tube and the rotational components via cables for operation. This type of generator was mounted on the rotational component of the CT system and rotated with the X-ray tube. Some generators remain mounted inside the gantry wall. Some newer scanner designs utilize a generator that is located outside the gantry. Slip ring technology eliminated the need for cables and allows continuous rotation of the gantry components without interference of cables.

X-ray tubes: CT procedures facilitate the use of large exposure factors, (high mA and KvP values) and short exposure times. A typical spiral/helical CT scan of the abdomen may require the continuous production of X-rays for a 30 to 40 second period. CT systems produce X-radiation continuously or in short millisecond bursts or pulses at high mA and kVp values. CT X-ray tubes must possess a high heat capacity which is the amount of heat that a tube can store without operational damage to the tube. The X-ray tube needs the design which will absorb high heat levels generated from the high speed rotation of the anode and the bombardment of electrons upon the anode surface. An X-ray tubes heat capacity is expressed in heat units. Modern CT systems utilize X-ray tubes that have a heat capacity of approximately 2 to 7 million heat units (MHU) with cooling rates as fast as 1 mhu/min. A CT X-ray tube must also possess a high heat dissipation rate. Many CT X-ray tubes utilize a combination of oil and air cooling systems to eliminate heat and maintain continuous operation. Early generations CT scanners used fixed anode, oil cooled X-ray tubes which had fairly limited capabilities. Recent X-ray tubes use rotating graphite anode with unique cooling system. This type of X-ray tube anode has a large diameter with graphite backing which allows it to absorb and dissipate large amounts of heat. The focal spot size of an X-ray tube is determined by the size of the filament and cathode which is determined by the manufacturer. Most X-ray tubes have more than one focal spot size. The use of a small focal spot increases detail but it concentrates heat onto a smaller portion of the anode therefore, more heat is generated. CT tubes utilize a bigger filament than conventional radiography X-ray tubes which increases the size of the effective focal spot. Decreasing the anode or target angle decreases the size of the effective focal spot. The anode angle of a conventional radiography tube is usually between 12° and 17°, while CT tubes employ a target angle approximately between 7° and 10°. The decreased anode or target angle also helps alleviate some of the effects caused by the heel effect. CT can compensate any loss of resolution to due to the use of larger focal spot sizes by employing resolution enhancement algorithms such as bone or sharp algorithms, targeting techniques and decreasing section thickness.

Collimation: In CT collimation of the X-ray beam includes tube or source collimators, a set of pre-patient collimators and post-patient or pre-detector collimators. The tube or source collimators are located in the X-ray tube and determine the section thickness that will be utilized for a particular CT scanning procedure. When the CT technician selects a section thickness he or she is determining tube collimation by narrowing or widening the beam. A second set of collimators located directly below the tube collimators maintain the width of the beam as it travels toward the patient. A final set of collimators called post-patient or predetector collimators are located below the patient and above the detector. The primary responsibilities of this set of collimators are to insure proper beam width at the detector and reduce the number of scattered photons that may enter a detector.

Filtration: There are two types of filtration utilized in CT, Inherent tube Filtration and Mathematical filters. Inherent tube filtration and filters made of aluminum or Teflon are utilized in CT to shape the beam intensity by filtering out low energy photons that contribute to the production of scatter. Special filters called "bow-tie" filters absorb low energy photons before reaching the patient. Ideal X-ray beam should be monochromatic or composed of photons having the same energy. However, in practice the X-ray beams are polychromatic in nature containing photons of much different energy.

Heavy filtration of the X-ray beam results in a more uniform beam. The more uniform the beam, the more accurate the attenuation values or CT numbers are for the scanned anatomical region. Mathematical filters such as bone or soft tissue algorithms are included into the CT reconstruction process to enhance resolution of a particular anatomical region of interest.

Data acquisition systems: These are the heart of CT scanner and have three main components-The detector system, Analog-to-digital conversion and some data preprocessing for use by scanner reconstruction system. These convert X-ray flux to electric current, electric current to voltage and analog voltage to digital form. It subtracts background offset signals, provides logarithmic conversion of data and transmits data to preprocessing system.

Detectors: When the X-ray beam travels through the patient, it is attenuated by the anatomical structures it passes through. In conventional radiography, we utilize a film-screen system as the primary image receptor to collect the attenuated information. The CT process relies on collecting attenuated photon energy and converting it to an electrical signal, which is then converted to a digital signal for computer reconstruction. The image receptors that are utilized in CT are referred to as detectors. A detector is a crystal or ionizing gas that when struck by an X-ray photon produces light or electrical energy. The two types of detectors utilized in CT systems are scintillation or solid state and xenon gas detectors. Scintillation detectors utilize a crystal that fluoresces when struck by an X-ray photon which produces light energy. A photodiode which transforms the light energy into electrical or analog energy is attached to the scintillation portion of the detector. The strength of the detector signal is proportional to the number of attenuated photons that are successfully converted to light energy and then to an electrical or analog signal. The signal represents an absorption or attenuation profile which is obtained for each view or projection and every detector in the detector array is responsible for this task. The most frequently used scintillation crystals are made of Bismuth Germinate and Cadmium Tungstate. Earlier Sodium and Cesium Iodide were utilized as the light producing agent, however at times they would fluoresce more than necessary and the afterglow problems associated with them altered the strength of the detector signal which could cause in accuracies during computer reconstruction.

The second type of detector utilized for CT imaging system is a gas detector, usually constructed utilizing a chamber made of a ceramic material with long thin ionization plates made of tungsten acting as electron collection plates submerged in xenon gas. When attenuated photons interact with the charged

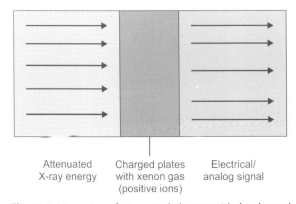

| Attenuated X-ray energy | Charged plates with xenon gas (positive ions) | Electrical/analog signal |

Fig. 13.1 Interaction of attenuated photons with the charged plates with the xenon gas ionization producing an electrical current

plates and the xenon gas ionization of ions occurs producing an electrical current (Fig. 13.1). Xenon gas is the element of choice because of it remains stable under extreme amounts of pressure. Xenon detectors use high pressure (about 25 atmospheres) gas between two ionization plates. Utilization of more gas in a detector increases the number of molecules that can be ionized increasing the strength of the detector signal or response. The long thin tungsten plates of the gas detector are highly directional and ionization of the plates and the resultant detector signal rely on attenuated photons entering the chamber and ionizing the gas. If the xenon gas detectors are not positioned properly the ability of the detector to produce an accurate signal is compromised because the photons may miss the chamber. The xenon gas detectors are generally fixed with the position of the X-ray tube seen with 3rd generation scanner geometry designs. Because of their high directionality xenon detectors cannot be used in fourth-generation CT.

Detector efficiency describes the percent of incoming photons that a detector converts to a useable electrical signal. The two primary factors that determine how well a detector can capture photons relative to efficiency are the width and the distance between each detector. It is important that detectors are placed as close to one another as possible. Scintillation detectors convert 99 to 100% of the attenuated photons into a useable electrical signal. Xenon gas detectors are less efficient, converting 60 to 90% of the photons that enter the chambers due to compromised efficiency because of absorption of some of the photons by the ionization plates. Also, photons may pass through the chamber without interacting with the gas molecules. One advantage to this situation may be the low scatter acceptability as some of the photons absorbed by the plates are scattered photons and as in conventional radiography scatter also adversely affects the CT image. Scintillation detectors convert almost all the received information including scattered photons and have high scatter acceptability. The dynamic range determines the ability of a detector to detect and differentiate a wide range of X-ray intensities. By definition, dynamic range of a detector describes the range of X-ray exposures at the detector to which the system can respond without saturation and produce satisfactory gray-scale images. Current CT systems have an approximate dynamic range of 1,000,000 to 1 and 1,100 views or projections a second meaning that CT systems have the ability to respond to 1,000,000 X-ray intensities at approximately 1,100 views per second which is beyond the display systems and human visual perception limits.

CT patient table or couch: The final component of the scan or imaging system is the patient table or couch. CT tables or couches need to be made of a material that will not cause artifacts when scanned for example carbon fiber material. The movement of the table or couch is referred to as incrementation or indexing. Helical CT table incrementation or indexing is quantified in millimeters per second (mm/sec) because the table is moving for the entire scan. All table or couch designs have weight limits that if exceeded may compromise incrementation or indexing accuracy. Various attachments are available for different types of scanning procedures.

Development of CT: The development of the first modern CT scanner was begun in 1967 by Godfrey Hounsfield, an engineer at British EMI Corp. Hounsfield was interested in situations in which large amounts of potential information may be efficiently used. He estimated that by taking careful measurements of X-ray transmission through a subject at many positions across the subject and at a sufficient number of angles, it should be possible to determine attenuation differences of 0.5% which could possibly be sufficient to distinguish between soft tissues. After verification of his hypothesis with a laboratory apparatus, the first clinical CT scanner (original EMI Mark I first-generation CT scanner) was built and installed at Atkinson-Morley Hospital in England in September 1971. Both conspicuity and contrast could be improved if irradiation and visualization were limited to individual cross-sectional imaged slices, which could be displayed as 2-dimensional images without significant structure overlap. Because the radiation source could be collimated to thin (1 cm) slices, significantly less scatter would be generated (because less tissue would be irradiated at any given time). One way to achieve this goal is the process of reconstruction from projections. Interestingly, the theory of image reconstruction from projections, which is central to the basic concept of CT, was described in 1917 and was proposed for medical imaging as early as 1940.

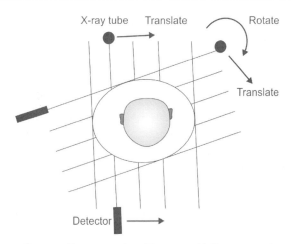

Fig. 13.2 First generation CT system with linear scan of source and detector—rotate/translate, pencil beam scan

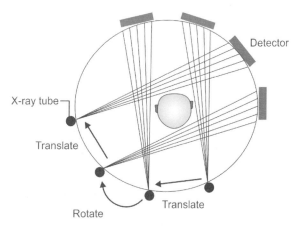

Fig. 13.3 Second generation CT system—rotate/translate, narrow fan beam with X-ray head and detectors mounted onto C-arm frame that could rotate 180°

First generation CT system (rotate/translate, pencil beam): The earliest First generation CT scanners were designed to acquire CT images of the patient's head and were based on parallel-beam geometry with translate-rotate principle of tube and detector combination (Fig. 13.2). These scanners used a thin slit X-ray beam and single X-ray detector to acquire the entire CT image. The X-ray head and detector were mounted on a C-arm frame and onto a synchronized linear scan mechanism that could be rotated through an arc of 180°. The C-arm would be rotated into position stopped and held still while the linear scanning mechanism moved the thin slit X-ray beam across the anatomical view. Small detector monitored the intensity of beam before entering body to yield value of incident intensity (I_0). Each linear scan produced one view or X-ray image. The C-arm would be positioned in 1° steps to allow 180 linear scans along the 180° arc. The linear scan mechanism allowed 240 detector measurements at 1.7 mm intervals to create each of the 180 views. Some scanners had two X-ray beams and a second detector to allow the scanner to acquire two anatomical section scans at the same time. A complete CT scan and image reconstruction took upto 10 minutes. The disadvantages were long scanning time and compromised image quality due to patient motion.

Second generation system (rotate/translate, narrow fan beam): A fan shaped X-ray beam (3–10° diverging angle) was projected onto a linear array of approximately 30 detectors. The X-ray head and detectors were mounted onto a C-arm frame that could rotate 180° around the patient (Fig. 13.3). The increased number of detectors reduced the number of linear scans required during the 180° arc, reducing the time required for a scan to less than 90 seconds. Reduced scan times allowed the patient to hold their breath for the entire scan allowing

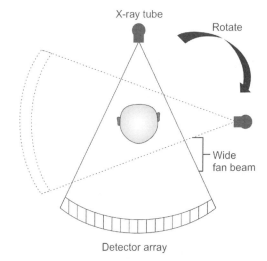

Fig. 13.4 Third generation CT system—rotate/rotate, wide fan beam—An arc of detectors and X-ray tube rotate continuously around patient for 360°

the radiographer to scan the thoracic region of the body. The fan shaped beam increased scatter radiation artifact forcing the use of lead masks on the detectors to reduce this scatter radiation artifact.

Third generation system (rotate/rotate, wide fan beam): A wider fan shaped X-ray beam (50 to 55°) and a curved array of 250 to 750 detectors. The wider beam and larger detector array allowed the scanner to include the entire body in a single exposure. An arc of detectors and X-ray tube rotate continuously around patient for 360° eliminating the need for linear scanning to be combined with the X-ray head rotation (Fig. 13.4). Third generation scanners would acquire approximately 700,000 measurements per anatomical section. Scan times reduced to less than 12 seconds. Shorter scan times allowed sequential scans to approximated dynamic functions with approximately

4 scans per minute. In this configuration detectors are fixed radially and do not view scan areas uniformly with only center detectors in arc see the pixels at center of field of view (FOV). However, this fixed relationship allows detectors to be highly collimated reducing scatter radiation and hence image noise. Spatial resolution, a key image parameter of CT depends on how closely spaced are detectors (number of detectors in an arc). Number of detectors in arc ranges from, 600 to more than 900, limiting spatial resolution to 5 to 10 line pairs per centimeter. However, the single detector array made third generation scanners prone to ring artifact.

Fourth generation system (rotate/stationary): A single projection wide angle fan shaped X-ray beam (50 to 55°) and fixed detector arc with 600 to 2000 stationary detectors. The detectors are fixed in a circular ring around the patient and X-ray head and alignment of the X-ray beam to each detector is essential (Fig. 13.5). The X-ray head travels more than 360° in order to provide an acceleration and deceleration zone. Scanning takes place as the X-ray head travels in either direction, clockwise and counter clockwise. Scan rates of approximately 15 scans per minute are achieved and are limited by the interscan time used to change the direction of the X-ray head travel. Dynamic scanning and overscanning modes using scanning arcs of greater than 360° are available. This geometry permits very high spatial resolution (more than 20 lines/cm). However there is increased detection of scattered radiation leading to image noise.

Fifth generation: Stationary/stationary, electron beam: A novel CT scanner was developed for cardiac tomographic imaging. This "cine CT" scanner does not use a conventional X-ray tube and is usually used in cardiology. A large ring that circles the patients is used which lies directly opposed to the detector ring. The

X-rays are produced from the focal track as a high—energy electron beam. There are no moving parts to this scanner gantry. The electron beam is produced in a vacuum pump. It is capable of 50-milisecond scan times and can produce 17 CT slices each second for example in heart structures.

Volume (spiral/helical) CT: Spiral CT design makes it possible to achieve greater rotational velocities than conventional systems, which allows for shorter scan time. The aim of spiral CT is to obtain meaningful CT data as patient move through rotating, continuous fan beam exposure. Instead of obtaining data sequentially during individual exposure; a block of data in the form of cork-screw or helix is obtained. If the table movement occurs at such a speed that during one revolution of tube patient is moved by distance equal to slice thickness complete volume of tissue is examined. Before advent of spiral CT, in third and fourth generation CT data is obtained in discrete slices of patient anatomy in a method commonly called as axial scanning. In axial scanning, each revolution of X-ray tube around patient produces single data set (slice). During data collection patient table is motionless. To create an additional slice, table is advanced to given amount and X-ray tube is once again rotated around the patient.

Advanced slip ring technology is used to allow the X-ray head to travel in one direction indefinitely. The X-ray head does not have to be decelerated and accelerated in between scans. Approximately 1000 detectors are aligned opposite the X-ray tube. The moving detector array travels in a circle around the patient at the same time as the X-ray head moves. The patient can be advanced through the CT gantry as the continuously revolving X-ray head circles the patient (Fig. 13.6). The computer acquires measurements from the detectors that result in data representing a continuous helical scan. The primary advantage to helical scans is the reduced scan time for example the entire abdomen can be scanned in single breath hold. This results in the use of less contrast media, less motion artifact and greater patient through put. The primary disadvantage is that the entire 360° scan information is not acquired for every anatomical cross section. Computer reconstruction is required to fill in the missing data. Three key advances enable CT data to be acquired continuously with ongoing patient movement—Slip-ring technology, precise patient table transport, Software reconstruction algorithms.

Slip-ring technology: In conventional CT systems, there was inherent delay of 3 to 5 sec between each exposure which arose from physical need to have cables connecting stationary gantry and rotating tube-detector assembly. After 1 to 3 exposure, depending

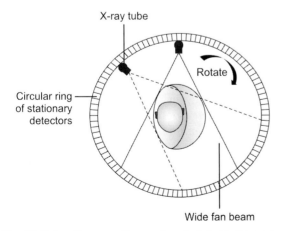

Fig. 13.5 Fourth generation system (rotate/stationary)—detectors are fixed in circular ring around the patient and X-ray head which travels more than 360°

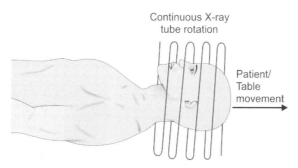

Fig. 13.6 Volume (spiral/helical) CT—X-ray tube rotates continuously and the patient moves through the X-ray beam at a constant rate

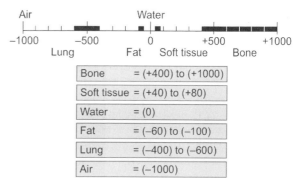

Fig. 13.7 The Hounsfield scale of CT numbers

on cable length, the cable become wound and then rotation of tube-detector assembly had to stop, change direction to unwind. Slip-ring technology abolished the physical need for presence of electric cable between generator and moving tube-detector assembly. In this power from generator is connected to large stationary ring and other large ring that house the X-ray-detector assembly moves around within stationary ring. Power is transmitted between stationary and moving ring by means of brushes making it possible to have continuous X-ray tube rotation (rather than back and forth) and continuous data acquisition.

Multislice spiral CT: All multislice spiral CT system use third generation geometry with added dimension of multiple arcs of detectors. The first deployment of this technology include dual-arc detector in which two parallel arcs of detectors are used to simultaneously acquire data during single revolution of scan frame dividing total X-ray beam into two equal beams.

Analog-to-digital conversion: Once the detector generates the analog or electrical signal it is directed to the data acquisition system (DAS). The analog signal generated by the detector is a weak signal and must be amplified to be further analyzed which is done by the data acquisition system (DAS). The DAS is located in the gantry right after or above the detector system, however, in some modern CT scans the signal amplification occurs within the detector itself. The projection or raw data is in the form of an electrical or analog signal is first converted to digital information before sending to the computer. This task is accomplished by an analog to digital converter which is an essential component of the DAS. The digital signal is transferred to an array processor which solve solves the statistical information using algorithmic calculations essential for mathematical reconstruction of a CT image. Reconstruction is conversion of digital data provided by data acquisition system to a form that is suitable for viewing on viewing monitor. An array processor is a specialized high speed computer designed to execute mathematical

algorithms for the purpose of reconstruction and solves reconstruction mathematics faster than a standard microprocessor. Special algorithms may require several seconds to several minutes for a standard microprocessor to compute. Recently, processors termed as image or reconstruction generator that compute CT reconstruction mathematics faster than an array processors have been utilized to solve reconstruction mathematics essential to the development of CT fluoroscopy.

For each ray projection measurement made during CT scan, fundamental equation ($I = I_0 e^{-mx}$) is generated and complete set of such equations must then be solved to obtain individual value of 'm' for each matrix element. Many methods have been devised to solve set of equations generated in scan of which commonly used is *filtered back-projection* method. To eliminate blurring filtering or convolution "kernel" is used. Two types of filters or kernels used are—smooth (low frequency) filter to examine soft tissue and edge enhancement (high frequency) filter to examine bone. *CT number scale:* CT number is linear attenuation coefficient of X-rays, is given by,

$$CT\ number = \frac{K\,(M\text{-}Mw)}{Mw}$$

Where,
Mw-attenuation coefficient of water
M-attenuation coefficient of pixel in question.
K-1000 (original EMI scanner used value of 500)

In honour of Godfrey Hounsfield, CT unit is called a *Hounsfield unit (HU).* Air has value of (–)1000 *HU,* water 0 *HU,* bone +1000 *HU* (Fig. 13.7).

WINDOW SETTINGS

Window width: Window width is the range of CT numbers selected for grey scale.
Window level: Window level is the central CT number that determines position of window on HU scale. A narrow window would have sharper contrast. Wide

window would have greater latitude. The choice of window is determined by range of CT numbers to be investigated. For example, investigation of hemorrhage requires narrow window and investigation of middle ear disease needs wide window. As a general rule, the human eye can not appreciate contrast differences of less than 10%, whereas CT scanners can easily demonstrate differences of less than 1%. Therefore, small density resolution difference measured by CT scanners must be exaggerated to permit viewing. This can be done by selecting small range of gray scale. For example, CT number of liver tissue range is between 40 to 90 HU.

TYPICAL DOSES FOR COMPUTED TOMOGRAPHY

Dose is a measure of radiation risk. The radiation dose delivered during a CT scan is somewhat greater than that administered for an equivalent radiographic image. However, because the radiation is distributed quite homogeneously in a CT scan and the volume of the irradiated tissue is different with each slice a straight dose between a CT scan and a radiographic procedure is misleading. Probably, the better is an integral dose. Integral dose is a measure of the amount of energy deposited in tissue.

Integral dose (joules) = Dose (joules/kg) × Mass of irradiated tissue (kg)

Scan Type	Slice Thickness	Dose
Head	10 mm	65 mGy (6.5 Rads)
Spine	5 mm	23 mGy (2.3 Rads)
Body	10 mm	15–25 mGy (1.5–2.5 Rads)

COMPUTED TOMOGRAPHY IMAGE QUALITY

The most important functions of a computed tomography (CT) system is to reproduce a three dimensional structure and represent that structure as an accurate two-dimensional cross-section image. Spatial resolution, contrast resolution, linearity, noise and artifacts are the primary characteristics that effect image quality in CT. Enhancing or suppressing any of these characteristics depends upon the imaging interests and the region of the body being scanned. The changing CT parameters such as section thickness, algorithms and field of view also have a significant effect on the overall quality of the CT image. CT image quality is dependent upon balancing these characteristics and parameters to produce the best possible image for the anatomical region being scanned. Image noise and artifacts are the two biggest problem of CT image quality. CT parameters can be manipulated to either

decrease or eliminate the adverse effects of these image quality characteristics. For example, if a bone reconstruction algorithm is utilized to increase spatial resolution, image noise increases which degrades contrast or soft tissue resolution. Increasing technical factors such as mAs or kVp decreases image noise but an increase in patient dose occurs. Hence the goal is to manipulate CT parameters according the imaging interest or situation with aim to maintain minimum possible patient radiation dose.

IMAGE ARTIFACTS

Streak and ring artifacts: Detector miscalibration in 3rd generation scanner leads to ring artifacts. Poor alignment of tube and detector causes blurring of edge or ring or streak artifact. Detectors in center of arc are most sensitive for causing these artifacts. Fourth generation scanner are more prone to cause streak artifacts.

Metal and bone artifact: The objects of exceptionally high or low HU can cause artifacts by forcing detectors to operate in a nonlinear response region. For example, metal pin and gas can produce streak artifact. The range of X-ray intensity values to which scanner can accurately respond is called the dynamic range. Larger the dynamic range less prone is instrument for such artifact.

Beam hardening artifact: Beam hardening artifacts results from preferential absorption of low energy photon from beam. Examples are shadow beneath rib, Inter-petrous streaking.

Partial volume artifact: When tissues of widely varying attenuation properties occupy same voxel, then attenuation of voxel is equal to average attenuation of two tissues.

Motion artifact: These are usually streak or sunburst type of artifacts occurring where there is high or low density interface (for example bowel gas) and patient motion during scan.

Stair-stepping artifact: In x-y plane direction, the pixel of reformatted image has same length as axial image and in z axis pixel length is equal to slice thickness. Since in most scans, pixel length is much smaller than slice thickness, the reformatted scans show unusual appearance of stair-stepping artifact.

Spiral pitch artifact: Spiral pitch artifacts are seen because larger pitch factor used to attain maximum coverage. Star pattern is seen in multislice CT where numbers of spokes of star are directly related to number of multislice detector row.

Cone beam artifact: As number of rows in multislice increases, the divergence of con beam along z-axis becomes significant. This should be rectified using reconstruction process.

14

Magnetic Resonance Imaging

Manisha Hadgaonkar

HISTORY

Magnetic resonance imaging (MRI) is the most important diagnostic imaging discovery in medicine since the discovery of X-ray in 1895 by Wilhelm Conrad Roentgen. The first MRI was commercially available in 1980. Since then its importance in field of medicine continues to grow at a tremendous space and is now established beyond doubt. Before beginning a study, it is important to know a brief history of MRI.

Sir Joseph Larmor (1857–1942) developed the equation that the angular frequency of precession of the nuclear spins being proportional to the strength of the magnetic field referred as Larmor relationship. In the 1930's, Isidor Isaac Rabi of Columbia University succeeded in detecting and measuring single states of rotation of atoms and molecules, and in determining the magnetic and mechanical moments of the nuclei.

Working independently, Felix Bloch of Stanford University and Edward Purcell of Harvard University made the first successful nuclear magnetic resonance experiment to study chemical compounds in 1946, thus magnetic resonance phenomenon was discovered. They developed instruments, which could measure the magnetic resonance in bulk material such as liquids and solids. 1946 they came up with the idea to use magnets to take pictures of a living being and called it magnetic resonance. Both Felix Bloch and Edward Purcell were awarded Nobel Prize in 1952.

In 1971, Raymond Damadian a physician and scientist of State University of New York demonstrated that there are different T1 relaxation times between normal and abnormal tissues of the same type, as well as between different types of normal tissues on his Nuclear Magnetic Resonance (NMR) device. In the same year he proved that magnetic resonance could be used to help detect diseases by the different nuclear magnetic relaxation times between tissues and tumors thus motivating scientists to consider magnetic resonance for the detection of disease.

In 1973, Paul Christian Lauterbur (6 May 1929– 27 March 2007) of State University of New York described a new imaging technique that he termed Zeugmatography. By utilizing gradients in the magnetic field, this technique was able to produce a two-dimensional image. Magnetic resonance imaging was first demonstrated on small test tube samples. He used a back projection technique similar to that used in CT.

In 1975, Richard Ernst introduced 2-Dimentional NMR using phase and frequency encoding, and Fourier Transformer instead of Paul Lauterbur's back-projection, he timely switched magnetic field gradients. This basic reconstruction method is the basis of current MRI techniques.

On 3 July 1977 Raymond Damadien performed the first MRI examination on a human being on the machine which he named "Indomitable." It took four hours and 45 minutes to complete.

Peter Mansfield further developed the utilization of gradients in the magnetic field and the mathematical analysis of these signals for a more useful imaging technique. 1977 the first images taken of a cross section through a finger were presented by Peter Mansfield and Andrew Maudsley. Peter Mansfield also could present the first image through the abdomen. In the same year Peter Mansfield developed the echo planar imaging (EPI) technique. This technique developed in later years to produce images at video rates (30 ms/image). Paul Lauterbur and Peter Mansfield were awarded with the Nobel Prize in Medicine in 2003.

Raymond Damadien in 1978 founded the FONAR Corporation, which manufactured the first commercial MRI scanner in 1980. As late as 1982, there were a handful of MRI scanners in the world. Today there are a million or even more, and images can be created in seconds what used to take hours. Current MRI scanners produce highly detailed 2-dimensional and 3-dimensional images. The technique was initially called nuclear magnetic resonance imaging (NMR or NMRI) but because of the negative connotations associated with the word nuclear it is called as magnetic resonance imaging.

PHYSICS

Magnetic resonance (MR) imaging is based on the electromagnetic activity of atomic nuclei. The human body is made up of more than 80% of water which contains hydrogen and oxygen atoms. Atomic nuclei are made up of protons and neutrons, both of which have spins. The hydrogen nucleus with atomic number 1 contains one proton and one electron. The proton is positively charged and acts like a tiny bar magnet. This H^1 particle is the most important in MRI because it is in abundance in the human body and also it has the highest gyro magnetic ratio. Those nuclei which have odd number of protons have a net spin and are thus magnetically active nuclei. Other nuclei for example, fluorine (19F) is magnetically active nuclei nuclei and may be used.

Each nucleus rotates around its own axis. As the nucleus spins, its motion induces a magnetic field when the nuclei are exposed to an external magnetic field (B_0), the interaction of the magnetic fields (i.e. the fields of the spinning nuclei and the externally applied field) causes the nuclei to wobble, or precess. The frequency at which precession occurs is defined by the Larmor equation.

Larmor equation is $\omega_0 = B_0 \times \gamma$

Where ω_0 is the precessional frequency, B_0 is the external magnetic field strength (measured in teslas), and γ is the gyromagnetic ratio (measured in megahertz per tesla), which is a constant for every atom at a particular magnetic field strength.

Until the hydrogen nuclei are exposed to B_0 magnetization (external magnetic field), their axis are randomly aligned. However, when B_0 magnetization is applied, the magnetic axis of the nuclei align with the magnetic axis of B_0, some in parallel and others in opposition to it (Fig. 14.1).

The cumulative effect of all the magnetic moments of the nuclei is the net magnetization vector.

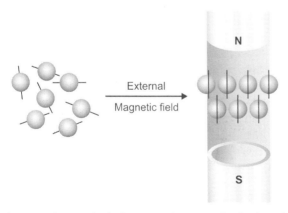

Fig. 14.1 The axis the hydrogen nuclei are randomly aligned but when B_0 magnetization is applied, the magnetic axes of the nuclei align with the magnetic axis of B_0

When a radiofrequency (RF) pulse is applied, the RF excitation causes the net magnetization vector to flip by a certain angle and this produces two magnetization vector components, longitudinal magnetization and transverse magnetization.

As the transverse magnetization processes around a receiver coil, it induces a current in that coil, in accordance with the Faraday law of induction. This current becomes the MR signal.

When the RF energy source is turned off, the net magnetization vector realigns with the axis of B_0 through the process of T1 recovery, during which longitudinal magnetization increases in magnitude, or recovers. At the same time, the transverse magnetization decreases (decays) through additional mechanisms known as T2*decay and T2 decay. Different tissues have different T1, T2, and T2* values. Furthermore, T2* is dependent on the magnetic environment (the spatial uniformity of the external field).

Fat has a shorter T1 (i.e. recovers faster) and a shorter T2 (i.e. decays faster) than water, which has a relatively long T1 and T2. T2* decay occurs very quickly in both fat and water.

During T1 (spin-lattice) relaxation, the longitudinal magnetization recovers as the spinning nuclei release energy into the environment. During T2 (spin-spin) relaxation, the transverse magnetization is dephased because of interaction between the spinning nuclei and their magnetic fields. In T2* signal decay, the transverse magnetization is dephased because of magnetic field in-homogeneities. The magnetic field is not exactly the same everywhere; in some places, it is a bit stronger ($B_0 + \alpha$) for example, 1.505 T—and in others it is a bit weaker ($B_0 - \alpha$) for example, 1.495 T. Such differences may occur because of the presence of metallic objects, air, dental implants, or calcium, or they may be due to the limitations of magnet construction.

At MR imaging, differences in T1, T2, and proton density, i.e. the number of H nuclei in various tissues create differences in tissue contrast on images. Two key parameters-repetition time (TR) and echo time (TE) are key to the creation of image contrast. It is important to recognize these symbols, because they are invariably used to represent TR and TE.

TR is the time (usually measured in milliseconds) between the application of an RF excitation pulse and the start of the next RF pulse.

TE measured in milliseconds is the time between the application of the RF pulse and the peak of the echo detected. Both parameters affect contrast on MR images because they provide varying levels of sensitivity to differences in relaxation time between various tissues.

At short TRs, the difference in relaxation time between fat and water can be detected (longitudinal magnetization recovers more quickly in fat than in water); at long TRs, it cannot be detected. Therefore, TR relates to T1and affects contrast on T1-weighted images. At short TEs, Differences in the T2 signal decay in fat and water cannot be detected; at long TEs, they can be detected. Therefore, TE relates to T2 and affects contrast on T2-weighted images.

Tissue Contrast: All MR images are affected by each of the parameters that determine tissue contrast, i.e. T1, T2, and proton density, but the TR and TE can be adjusted to emphasize a particular type of contrast. This may be done, for example, with T1 weighting. In T1-weighted MR imaging, while the images show all types of contrast, T1 contrast is accentuated. Table 14.1 describes the parameters used to obtain images with T1, T2, and proton-density weighting. T1-weighted images best depict the anatomy and, if contrast material is used, they also may show pathologic entities; however, T2-weighted images provide the best depiction of disease, because most tissues that are involved in a pathologic process have higher water content than normal, and the fluid causes the affected areas to appear bright on T2-weighted images. Proton-density weighted MR images usually depict both the anatomy and the disease entity. The levels of signal intensity that characterize various tissues on T1- and T2-weighted images are shown in Table 14.2.

Table 14.1 Effect of time to repetition (TR) and time to echo (TE) for MR sequences on image contrast

Imaging technique	TR (time to repetition)	TE (time to echo)
T1-weighting or T1W	Short	Short
T2-weighting or T2W	Long	Long
Proton density weighting or PDW	Long	Short

Table 14.2 Signal intensity of various tissues at T1, T2 and proton density imaging

Tissue	T1	T2	Proton density
Fat	Bright	Bright (less than T1)	Bright
Water	Dark	Bright	Intermediate bright
Cerebral gray matter	Gray	Gray	Gray
Cerebral white matter	White	Dark	Dark
TR values	TR < 500	TR > 1500	TR > 1500
TE values	TE 50 to 100	TE > 80	TE < 50

MAGNETIC RESONANCE SIGNAL LOCALIZATION

Magnetic resonance imaging detects the signal from the respective tissue by means of employing gradient.

Gradients are linear variations of the magnetic field strength in a selected region. Along with the magnetic field strength, the precessional frequency of H1 nuclei is also changed in the specific region. Three types of gradients are applied, according to the axis of imaging (x, y, or z axis).The section selective gradient selects the section to be imaged, i.e. the target of the RF excitation pulse. The phase-encoding gradient causes a phase shift in the spinning protons so that the MR imaging system computer can detect and encode the phase of the spin. The frequency-encoding gradient also causes a shift that helps the MR system to detect the location of the spinning nuclei. Once the MR system processor has information on the frequency and phase of each spin, it can compute the exact location and amplitude of the signal. That information is then stored in k-space. k-space is a matrix of voxels within which the raw imaging data are stored in the MR imaging system. The center of k-space contains information about gross form and tissue contrast, whereas the edges or periphery of k-space contain information about spatial resolution or in other words details and fine structures. The raw imaging data in k-space must be Fourier transformed to obtain the final image.

Applications of MR sequences: Pulse sequences are wave forms of the gradients and RF pulses applied in MR image acquisition. There are only two fundamental types of MR pulse sequences: Spin Echo (SE) and Gradient recalled echo (GRE). All other MR sequences are variations of these, with different parameters added on. MR pulse sequences can be either two-dimensional (2D), with one section acquired at a time, or three-dimensional (3D), with a volume of multiple sections obtained in a single acquisition.

In SE sequences, a 90° pulse flips the net magnetization vector into the transverse plane. As the spinning nuclei go through T1, T2, and T2*relaxation, the transverse magnetization is gradually dephased. A 180° pulse is applied at a time equal to one-half of TE to rephase the spinning nuclei. When the nuclei are again spinning in phase (at total TE), an echo is produced and read. Most conventional SE sequences are very long and therefore are not used frequently.

However, advances in MR imaging technology have enabled a reduction in acquisition time with the use of fast SE sequences.

As mentioned earlier, sequences that have a short TR and short TE are used to obtain T1-weighting. Those with a long TR and short TE result in proton-density weighting. When the TR is long and the TE is

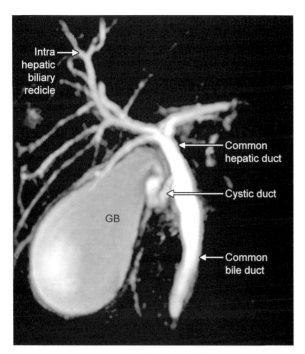

Fig. 14.2 MR cholangiography: Sagittal fast SE image with a heavily T2 weighted sequence

long, T2-weighting is achieved. Sequentially increasing the TE of a sequence weights it more heavily toward T2. This technique is used at MR cholangiography (Fig. 14.2) to obtain a detailed depiction of the bile ducts and pancreatic ducts.

Spin Echo based sequences: Fast SE Variants-In a fast or turbo SE sequence, a single 90° pulse is applied to flip the net magnetization vector, after which multiple 180° rephasing pulses are applied, each of which creates a Hahn echo. All the echoes together are called an echo train, and the total number of 180° RF pulses and echoes is referred to as the echo train length. The acquisition time is greatly reduced with use of a fast SE sequence as opposed to a conventional SE sequence. It is approximately proportional to 1/ETL, where ETL is the echo train length, for imaging of a single section or a small number of sections. However, at imaging of larger volumes, the reduction of acquisition time is highly dependent on the spatial coverage.

Conventional inversion recovery—This is a SE sequence in which a 180° preparatory pulse is applied to flip the net magnetization vector 180° and null the signal from a particular entity (e.g. water in tissue). When the RF pulse ceases, the spinning nuclei begin to relax. When the net magnetization vector for water passes the transverse plane (the null point for that tissue), the conventional 90° pulse is applied, and the SE sequence then continues as before. The interval between the 180° pulse and the 90° pulse is the TI. At TI, the net magnetization vector of water is very weak, whereas that for body tissues is strong. When the net magnetization vectors are flipped by the 90° pulse,

there is little or no transverse magnetization in water, so no signal is generated (fluid appears dark), whereas signal intensity ranges from low to high in tissues with a stronger net magnetization vector. Two important clinical implementations of the inversion recovery concept are the short TI inversion-recovery (STIR) sequence and the fluid-attenuated inversion-recovery (FLAIR) sequence.

SPECIAL SEQUENCES

- *Short Tau Inversion Recovery (STIR) Sequence:* It is heavily T2 weighted imaging, as a result the fluid and edema return high signal intensity and it annuls out the signal from fat. The resultant images show the areas of pathology clearly. The sequence is useful in musculoskeletal imaging as it annuls the signal from normal fatty bone marrow.
- *Fluid Attenuated Inversion Recovery (FLAIR):* This is an inversion-recovery pulse sequence that suppresses or annuls out the signal from fluid/CSF. The sequence is useful to show subtle lesions in the brain and spinal cord as it annuls the signal from CSF. It is useful to bring out the periventricular hyperintense lesions, e.g. in multiple sclerosis.
- *Gradient Echo Sequence:* This sequence reduces the scan times. This is achieved by giving a shorter RF pulse leading to a lesser amount of disruption to the magnetic vectors. The sequence is useful in identifying calcification and blood degradation products. Diffusion-Weighted Imaging 'Diffusion' portrays the movement of molecules due to random motion. It enables to distinguish between rapid diffusion of protons (unrestricted diffusion) and slow diffusion of protons (restricted diffusion). GRE pulse sequence has been devised to image the diffusion of water through tissues. It is a sensitive way of detecting acute brain infarcts, where diffusion is reduced or restricted.

FAST MAGNETIC RESONANCE IMAGING SEQUENCES

A number of fast MRI sequences have been proposed over the last two decades that greatly reduce the acquisition time either by repeatedly scanning the magnetization using a single excitation or by using multiple low flip-angle excitation schemes.

FLASH or SPGR

The word "spoiling" refers to the elimination of the steady-state transverse magnetization.

There are various ways of doing this, such as by applying RF spoiling, applying variable gradient spoilers and by lengthening TR. By eliminating the steady state component, only the longitudinal component affects the signal in the FLASH technique. This technique lends itself to reduced T2* weighting and increased T1-weighting. This is true provided that α is also large. When α is small, the T1 recovery curves play a minor role and proton density (PD) weighting is increased.

FISP (Fast Imaging with Steady-state Precession)

In contrast to spin echo (SE), in gradient echo (GRE) there may be residual transverse magnetization at the end of each cycle remaining for the next cycle. This residual magnetization reaches a steady state value after a few cycles. This residual steady state magnetization (MSS) is added to the transverse magnetization created by the next α RF Pulse and thus increases the length of the vector in the x-y plane. This then yields more T2* Weighting. In other words, tissues with a longer T2 have a longer MSS than do tissues with shorter T2. To preserve this steady state component, a "rewinder gradient" is applied in the Phase-encoding direction at the end of the cycle to reverse the effects of the Phase-encoding gradient applied at the beginning of the cycle.

PSIF (Reverse Fast Imaging with Steady-state Precession)

This technique yields heavily T2 weighted images. Each α pulse contains some 180º pulse embedded in it that acts like a refocusing pulse. This in turn will result in a spin echo at the time of the next α pulse. Hence, contrast is determined by T2 (not T2*).

Echo Planar Imaging

Single shot echo planar imaging (EPI) requires high performance gradients to allow rapid on and off switching of the gradients. The basic idea is to fill k-space in one shot with readout gradient during one T2* decay or in multiple shots (multishot EPI) by using multiple excitations. Single shot EPI allows oscillating frequency-encoding gradient pulses and complete k-space filling after a single RF pulse. Increased data processing speeds have allowed EPI to become clinically widespread and it is used in fMRI.

HASTE (Half-fourier Single-shot Turbo Spin Echo)

Half-fourier single-shot turbo spin echo (HASTE) is a single-shot version of the TSE technique. In this sequence, only slightly more than half the total number of required phase encoded lines of the k-space are acquired after one single RF excitation, which reduces scan time by nearly 2-fold compared with full k-space sampling. The rest of the k-space is filled by using the mirror symmetry of the k-space. However, the MR data have phase offsets that distort this symmetry. Therefore, a few extra lines near the center of k-space are acquired to calculate the phase correction. For example, to obtain an image of 128 or 256 matrix size, only 72 echoes are acquired, the first eight echoes are used to calculate the phase correction required for the half-Fourier reconstruction. HASTE image is then generated by taking the FT of the whole k-space data filled in this manner. The main advantage of using HASTE is its speed. Because it is a single-shot technique, an image can be obtained artifact free even without breath-hold. The insensitive nature of HASTE to patient movement and respiratory artifacts makes it very suitable for imaging uncooperative or pediatric patients. Disadvantages of using HASTE, on the other hand, include the significant image blurring due to T2 decay during the acquisition of multiple echoes, the high RF deposition due to the successive application of multiple 180° pulses and a lower SNR. HASTE sequences are widely used in clinical practice because of their speed and comparatively good image quality.

MAGNETIC RESONANCE ANGIOGRAPHY

Magnetic resonance angiography (MRA) is a group of techniques based on magnetic resonance imaging (MRI) to image blood vessels. Magnetic resonance angiography is used to evaluate arteries for stenosis, occlusion or aneurysms. MRA is often used to evaluate the arteries of the neck and brain, the thoracic and abdominal aorta, the renal arteries, and the legs. A variety of techniques can be used to generate the images, based on flow effects or on contrast. These images do not display the lumen of the vessel. They display the blood flowing through the vessel.

Flow Dependent Angiography

Flow dependent angiography (FDA) is based on blood flow. They take advantage of the fact that the blood within vessels is flowing to distinguish the vessels from other static tissue.

- Time-of-flight (TOF) or inflow angiography uses a short echo time and flow compensation to make flowing blood much brighter than stationary tissue. As flowing blood enters the area being imaged it has seen a limited number of excitation pulses so it is not saturated, this gives it a much higher signal than the saturated stationary tissue. As this method is dependent on flowing blood, areas with slow flow or flow that is in plane of the image may not be well visualized. This is most commonly used in the head and neck and gives detailed high-resolution images.

- *Phase-contrast (PC-MRA):* PC-MRA can be used to encode the velocity of moving blood in the magnetic resonance signals phase. The most common method used to encode velocity is the application of a bipolar gradient between the excitation pulse and the readout. A bipolar gradient is formed by two symmetric lobes of equal area.

Flow Independent Angiography

Flow independent angiography (FIA) rely on contrast agents (contrast enhanced techniques). These methods do not rely on flow. They are based on the differences of T1, T2 and chemical shift of the different tissues of the voxel.

- *Contrast enhanced (CE-MRA):* Injection of MRI contrast agents is currently the most common method of acquiring MRA. The contrast medium is injected into a vein, and images are acquired during the first pass of the agent through the arteries.
- *Non-contrast Enhanced Method:* These methods are based on the differences of T1, T2 and chemical shift of the different tissues of the voxel.

FUNCTIONAL MAGNETIC RESONANCE IMAGING

It is a relatively recent technique able to visualize cortical activity in patients in response to stimuli or actions. Functional magnetic resonance imaging (FMRI) is technically challenging to perform as the techniques used to visualize cortical activity (typically BOLD imaging) rely on minute changes in a low signal to noise ratio (SNR). Block testing design uses repeated blocks of activity (paradigm) separated by blocks of inactivity of alternative activity. This is by far the most frequently used study design in clinical fMRI. The activity performed or stimulus received by the patient is termed a paradigm, and each is designed to elicit a specific cortical response. In the clinical setting four paradigms suffice for most indications. These include visual, motor, speech and memory paradigm.

15

Computed Tomography Contrast Media

Hariqbal Singh

IODINATED INTRAVASCULAR AGENTS

Intravascular radiological contrast media are iodine containing chemicals which add to the details from any given CT scan study and thereby aid in the diagnosis. They were first introduced by Moses Swick. Iodine (atomic weight 127) is an ideal choice element for X-ray absorption because the korn (K) shell binding energy of iodine (33.7) is nearest to the mean energy used in diagnostic radiography and thus maximum photoelectric interactions can be obtained which are a must for best image quality. These compounds after intravascular injection are rapidly distributed by capillary permeability into extravascular-extracellular space and almost 90% is excreted via glomerular filtration by kidneys within 12 hours.

Following iodinated contrast media are available:

1. Ionic monomers, e.g. Diatrizoate, Iothamalate, Metrizoate.
2. Nonionic monomers, e.g. Iohexol, Iopamidol, Iomeron.

   Nonionic monomer contrast (Iohexol, Iopamidol or Iomeron) is a water-soluble radiographic contrast media. It is provided as a sterile, pyrogen-free, and colorless to pale-yellow solution sensitive to light and therefore should be protected from exposure. Its injection is hypertonic as compared to plasma and cerebrospinal fluid.

   Organic iodine compounds block X-rays as they pass through the body, thereby allowing body structures containing iodine to be delineated in contrast to those structures that do not contain iodine. The degree of opacity produced by these compounds is directly proportional to the total amount (concentration and volume) of the iodinated contrast agent in the path of the X-rays. After intrathecal administration into the subarachnoid space, diffusion of iohexol in the CSF allows the visualization of the subarachnoid spaces of the head and spinal canal. After intravascular administration, Nonionic contrast makes those vessels in its path of flow opaque, allowing visualization of the internal structures until significant hemodilution occurs.

   Uses: It is used intrathecally for myelography and in contrast enhancement for computerized tomography of head and body imaging. It is used for angiocardiography, aortography including aortic root, aortic arch, ascending aorta, abdominal aorta and branches; IV digital subtraction angiography of head, neck, abdominal, renal and peripheral vessels, peripheral arteriography and excretory urography, oral/ body cavity gastrointestinal (GI) tract, arthrography, hysterosalpingography (HSG).

   It is excreted mainly by renal system. In patients with impaired renal function, the elimination is prolonged depending upon the degree of impairment, thus, resulting in prolonged plasma levels of contrast.

   Patients sensitive to iodine may be sensitive to nonionic monomer contrast also. Adverse effects may vary directly with the concentration of the agent, the amount and technique used, and the underlying pathology. Increases in osmolality, volume, concentration, viscosity, and rate of administration of the solution may increase the incidence and severity of adverse effects. Most of the adverse effects are usually self-limited and of short duration. Overall incidence of adverse effects with nonionic contrast agents are less than with ionic contrast agents.

3. Ionic dimer, e.g. Ioxaglate.
4. Nonionic dimer, e.g. Iodixanol, Iotrolan.

The amount of contrast required is usually 1–2 mL/ kg body weight. Normal osmolality of human serum is 290 mOsm/kg. Ionic contrast media have much higher osmolality than normal human serum and are known as High Osmolar Contrast Media (HOCM), while nonionic contrast media have lower osmolality than normal human serum and are known as Low Osmolar Contrast Media (LOCM).

Following intravascular iodinated agent arterial opacification takes place at approximately 20 seconds with venous peak at approximately 70 seconds. The level then declines and the contrast is finally excreted by the kidneys. These different phases of enhancement are used to image various organs depending on the indication. Spiral CT, being faster is able to acquire images during each phase, thus provide much more information.

ORAL CONTRAST

The bowel is usually opacified in CT examinations of the abdomen and pelvis as the attenuation value of the bowel is similar to the surrounding structures and as a result pathological lesions can be obscured. Materials used include are barium or iodine based preparations, which are given the patient to drink preceding the examination to opacify the gastrointestinal tract.

Barium Sulfate

Barium sulfate preparations are used for evaluating gastrointestinal tract. Barium (atomic weight 137) is an ideal choice element for X-ray absorption because the K-shell binding energy of barium (37) is near to the mean energy used in diagnostic radiography and thus maximum photoelectric interactions can be obtained which are a must for best image quality. Moreover, barium sulfate is nonabsorbable, nontoxic and can be prepared into a stable suspension.

The barium crystals are made from milling of mineral barytes and precipitation with sulfuric acid. Barium sulfate is water insoluble and is available either as a powder or as a suspension. Large organic molecules, such as gum arabic, pectin and methyl carboxycellulose may be added to give the suspension good characteristics such as easy flow, good mucosal adhesion without cracking, high radiographic density in thin layers, and lack of foaming. Antifoaming agents may be added as well. The density of the suspension varies with the type of examination. Single-contrast Barium enemas require low-density suspensions, while double-contrast examinations of the stomach use medium or high-density suspensions.

Two main types of tests are conducted with the use of barium: the barium meal or barium swallow, for radiologic examination of the upper gastrointestinal tract, and the barium enema for examination of the lower gastrointestinal tract. They provide better delineation of mucosal details and are less expensive than water-soluble iodinated contrast media. The elimination rate is a function of gastrointestinal transit time. After GI application, it leaves the body with the feces. For CT scan of abdomen, 1000 to 1500 mL of 1 to 5% w/vol barium sulphate suspension can be used.

When intestinal perforation is suspected, a water-soluble iodinated contrast medium such as gastrografin may be used; when there is a possibility of aspiration, a nonionic water-soluble contrast medium is preferable.

Contraindications of barium sulfate products in case of known or suspected:
- Obstruction of the colon
- Gastrointestinal tract perforation
- Obstructing lesions of the small intestine
- Inflammation or neoplastic lesions of the rectum
- Hypersensitivity to barium sulfate formulations
- Recent rectal biopsy
- Pyloric stenosis.

Adverse reactions are rare. Rarely mediastinal leakage can lead to fibrosing mediastinitis while peritoneal leakage can cause adhesive peritonitis.

Iodinated Agents

Iodine containing oral contrast agents like Gastrografin and Trazograf are given for evaluating gastrointestinal tract on CT scan.

Air

Air is used as a negative per rectal contrast medium in large bowel during CT abdomen and during CT colonography.

Carbon Dioxide

Rarely carbon dioxide is used for infradiaphragmatic CT angiography in patients who are sensitive to iodinated contrast.

Adverse Reactions to Iodinated Contrast Media

Adverse reactions to iodinated contrast media (ICM) are classified as idiosyncratic and nonidiosyncratic.

Idiosyncratic Reactions

Idiosyncratic reactions typically begin within 20 minutes of the ICM injection, independent of the dose that is administered. A severe idiosyncratic reaction can occur after an injection of less than 1 mL of a contrast agent. Idiosyncratic reactions to ICM are called *anaphylactic reactions.*
- *Mild symptoms:* Mild symptoms include the following: scattered *urticaria*, which is the most commonly reported adverse reaction; *pruritus*; rhinorrhea; nausea, brief retching, and/or vomiting; diaphoresis; coughing; and *dizziness*. Patients with mild symptoms should be observed

for the progression or evolution of a more severe reaction, which requires treatment.

- *Moderate symptoms:* Moderate symptoms include the following: persistent vomiting; diffuse urticaria; *headache*; facial edema; laryngeal edema; mild bronchospasm or dyspnea; palpitations, tachycardia, or *bradycardia*; *hypertension*; and abdominal cramps.
- *Severe symptoms:* Severe symptoms include the following: *life-threatening arrhythmias* (i.e. *ventricular tachycardia*), *hypotension*, overt bronchospasm, laryngeal edema, *pulmonary edema, seizures, syncope*, and death.

Nonidiosyncratic Reactions

Nonidiosyncratic reactions include the following: bradycardia, hypotension, and *vasovagal reactions*; neuropathy; cardiovascular reactions; extravasation; and delayed reactions. Other nonidiosyncratic reactions include sensations of warmth, a metallic taste in the mouth, and nausea and vomiting.

- *Bradycardia, hypotension, and vasovagal reactions:* By inducing systemic parasympathetic activity, ICM can precipitate bradycardia and peripheral vasodilatation. The end result is systemic hypotension with bradycardia. This may be accompanied by other autonomic manifestations, including nausea, vomiting, diaphoresis, sphincter dysfunction, and mental status changes. Untreated, these effects can lead to cardiovascular collapse and death. Some vasovagal reactions may be a result of coexisting circumstances such as emotion, apprehension, pain, and abdominal compression, rather than ICM administration.
- *Nephropathy:* Contrast agent–related nephropathy is an elevation of the serum creatinine level that is more than 0.5 mg% or more than 50% of the baseline level at 1 to 3 days after the ICM injection. The elevation peaks by 3 to 7 days, and the creatinine level usually returns to baseline in 10 to 14 days. The incidence of contrast agent–related nephropathy in the general population is estimated to be 2 to 7%. As many as 25% of patients with this nephropathy have a sustained reduction in renal function, most commonly when the nephropathy is *oliguric*.

The mechanism of this type of nephropathy is thought to be a combination of pre-existing hemodynamic alterations; renal vasoconstriction, possibly through mediators such endothelin and adenosine; and direct ICM cellular toxicity. Patients with preexisting renal insufficiency have 5 to 10 times the risk of ICM-related nephropathy. Patients whose renal failure is the result of diabetic nephropathy are at the greatest risk. Azotemic diabetic patients also have the highest incidence of irreversible renal deterioration. In general, the higher the pre-existing serum creatinine level, the greater the likelihood of contrast agent–induced nephrotoxicity.

- *Cardiovascular reactions:* ICM can cause hypotension and bradycardia. Vasovagal reactions, a direct negative inotropic effect on the myocardium, and peripheral vasodilatation probably contribute to these effects. The latter 2 effects may represent the actions of cardioactive and vasoactive substances that are released after the anaphylactic reaction to the ICM. This effect is generally self-limiting, but it can also be an indicator of a more severe, evolving reaction.
- *Extravasation:* Extravasation of ICM into soft tissues during an injection can lead to tissue damage as a result of direct toxicity of the contrast agent or pressure effects, such as compartment syndrome.
- *Delayed reactions:* Delayed reactions become apparent at least 30 minutes after but within 7 days of the ICM injection. These reactions are identified in as many as 14 to 30% of patients after the injection of ionic monomers and in 8 to 10% of patients after the injection of nonionic monomers.

Common delayed reactions include the development of flulike symptoms, such as the following: fatigue, weakness, upper respiratory tract congestion, fevers, chills, nausea, vomiting, diarrhea, abdominal pain, pain in the injected extremity, rash, dizziness, and headache.

TREATMENT OF ADVERSE REACTIONS

Most acute severe adverse reactions to ICM occur within 20 minutes of injection. For this reason, the patient should be monitored for a minimum of 20 minutes after an ICM injection.

Rooms in which contrast material is administered should be stocked with appropriate basic and advanced life support monitoring equipment and drugs. The equipment should be regularly checked.

Principles of treatment of adverse reaction involves mainly five basic steps: ABCDE

A – Maintain proper airway.

B – Breathing – Support for adequate breathing.

C – Maintain adequate circulation. Obtain an IV access.

D – Use of appropriate drugs like antihistaminics for urticaria, atropine for vasovagal hypotension and bradycardia, beta agonists for bronchospasm, hydrocortisone, etc.

E – Always have emergency back-up ready including ICU care.

Treatment of Anaphylactic Reactions

A respiratory component to an adverse reaction requires more aggressive therapy. Oxygen administration, 10 to 12 L/min should be considered in any patient with respiratory difficulty. If bronchospasm is accelerating or severe, if it does not respond to inhalers, or if an upper airway edema (including laryngospasm) is present, epinephrine should be injected promptly. Intravenous use of epinephrine is optional in normotensive patients, but it is necessary in hypotensive patients with respiratory reactions.

H1 antihistamines, such as diphenhydramine, and H2-receptor blockers, such as cimetidine, do not have a major role in the treatment of respiratory reactions, but they may be administered after epinephrine.

Hypotension resulting from an anaphylactic reaction is treated with an intravenous iso-osmolar fluid (i.e. normal saline, Ringer lactate solution) in large volumes. Several liters of fluid may be required. If fluid and oxygen are unsuccessful in reversing the patient›s hypotension, the use of vasopressors should be considered. The most specifically effective vasopressor is dopamine; at infusion rates of 2 to 10 mcg/kg/min, the cerebral, renal, and splanchnic vessels remain dilated, whereas the peripheral vessels constrict. Epinephrine is less useful, its results are less predictable, and it has more adverse effects.

Urticaria

In asymptomatic patients, no treatment is needed.

In patient with symptomatic urticaria that is mild or moderate, diphenhydramine 50 mg may be administered intramuscularly, or intravenously.

In severe cases, treatment is as above; consider adding cimetidine 300 mg by slow intravenous injection or ranitidine 50 mg by slow intravenous injection.

Bronchospasm

For mild bronchospasm, treatment includes oxygen 10–12 L by face mask, close observation, and/or 2 puffs of an albuterol or metaproterenol inhaler.

For moderate cases without hypotension, treatment is as above, with epinephrine 1:1000, 0.1 to 0.3 mL given subcutaneously, repeated every 10 to 15 minutes as needed until 1 mL is administered.

In patients with severe bronchospasm, administer epinephrine 1:10,000 1 mL slow intravenous injection over approximately 5 minutes, repeated every 5 to 10 minutes as needed.

Laryngeal Edema

For mild to moderate laryngeal edema, treatment includes oxygen 10 to 12 L by face mask and epinephrine 1:1000 0.1 to 0.3 mL given subcutaneously, repeated every 10 to 15 minutes as needed until 1 mL is administered.

In moderate to severe cases, consider calling a code or intubating the patient. Consider adding diphenhydramine 50 mg slow intravenous injection and cimetidine 300 mg slow intravenous injection or ranitidine 50 mg slow intravenous injection.

Unresponsive Patient

In unresponsive patients, *defibrillation* may be needed to treat *ventricular fibrillation* and pulseless ventricular tachycardia.

Administer *basic life support*

Treatment of nonidiosyncratic reactions.

Extravasation Injuries

Extravasation injuries are treated by elevating the affected extremity and applying cold compresses. A plastic surgeon should be consulted if the patient's pain gradually increases over 2 to 4 hours, if skin blistering or ulceration develops, or if the circulation or sensation changes at or distal to the level of the extravasation. No specific treatment is unequivocally effective; therefore, most extravasation injuries are conservatively treated with supportive measures.

MAGNETIC RESONANCE IMAGING CONTRAST

Intravenous Contrast Agents

In magnetic resonance imaging (MRI), the most commonly used intravenous contrast agents are gadolinium chelates. The paramagnetic property of gadolinium provides contrast. It has the ability to alter the magnetic characteristics of neighboring tissues. The effect of this is shortening of the T1 and T2 relaxation times. Gadolinium containing contrast agents available are gadodiamide (Omniscan), gadobenic acid (Multihance), gadopentetic acid (Magnevist), gadoteridol (Prohance), gadofosveset (Ablavar), gadoversetamide (OptiMARK), gadoxetic acid (Eovist or Primovist).

MRI contrast agents are classified by the different changes in relaxation times after their injection:

- Positive contrast agents cause a reduction in the T1 relaxation time (increased signal intensity on T1 weighted images). They (appearing bright on MRI) are typically small molecular weight compounds containing as their active element Gadolinium, Manganese, or Iron. All of these elements have unpaired electron spins in their outer shells and long relaxivities. Some typical contrast agents as gadopentetate dimeglumine, gadoteridol, and gadoterate meglumine are utilized for the central nervous system and the complete body; mangafodipir trisodium is specially used for lesions of the liver and gadodiamide for the central nervous system.

- Negative contrast agents (appearing predominantly dark on MRI) are small particulate aggregates often termed superparamagnetic iron oxide (SPIO). These agents produce predominantly spin relaxation effects (local field inhomogeneities), which results in shorter T1 and T2 relaxation times. SPIO's and ultrasmall superparamagnetic iron oxides (USPIO) usually consist of a crystalline iron oxide core containing thousands of iron atoms and a shell of polymer, dextran, polyethylene glycol, and produce very high T2 relaxivities. USPIOs smaller than 300 nm cause a substantial T1 relaxation. T2 weighted effects are predominant. Available iron oxide contrast agents are Cliavist, Combidex, Resovist and Sinerem.

A special group of negative contrast agents (appearing dark on MRI) are perfluorocarbons (perfluorochemicals), because their presence excludes the hydrogen atoms responsible for the signal in MR imaging.

Hepatobiliary Contrast Agents

Hepatobiliary contrast agents are desirable for several reasons: to detect mass lesions such as metastases within the liver; to evaluate functional status of the liver in diffuse hepatocellular diseases such as cirrhosis; and to obtain high resolution images of the gallbladder and biliary tree.

Three advantages of a hepatobiliary contrast agent over a particulate agent targeted for Kupffer cells exist. First of all, there are many more hepatocytes than Kupffer cells (78% vs 2% by volume) in the liver, improving uptake efficiency of contrast material. Second, the biliary ducts are opacified by excreted contrast material, eliminating confusion of normal bile ducts from focal abnormalities as may occur with particulate agent contrast materials. Third, the contrast agent is rapidly excreted from the body reducing potential toxicity. In contrast, materials phagocytized by the reticuloendothelial system (including Kupffer cells) remain in the body for a long period of time.

- Manganese chloride ($MnCl_2$) is a prototype hepatobiliary contrast agent. IV and oral administration in animals results in a rapid decrease in the T1 relaxation time of the liver, spleen, kidneys, heart, and bile causing a bright signal on T1-weighted images. In its ionic state, Mn + 2, it is relatively toxic. Mn can be used in the form of a chelate with diminished toxicity for hepatobiliary imaging in humans.

- Chelates used as hepatobiliary contrast agents consist of a paramagnetic ion bound to an organic ligand, forming a complex that shows affinity for hepatocytes. This type of complex is desirable to increase uptake of the contrast agent by the hepatocytes and to reduce toxicity of the paramagnetic metal ion as is done with gadolinium. Possible chelates for hepatobiliary imaging include Fe-EHPG and derivatives, Gd-HIDA, Cr-HIDA, B-19036, and Mn-DPDP.

Magnetic Resonance Angiography (MRA)

All pulse sequences are sensitive to flow. There is a complex relationship between the type and rate of flow and the resultant signal intensity. As a general rule, fast or turbulent vascular flow results in a signal dropout, whilst slow vascular flow results in high signal. There are two principal flow sensitive sequences, time of flight and phase contrast. MRA can also be performed with intravenous gadolinium whilst in the vascular phase of enhancement.

Adverse Reactions of MRI Contrast Media

- *Minor side effects:* These are mild and temporary in nature. They include pain or burning at the injection site, low blood pressure, minor skin rash, mild headaches, blood clots, lightheadedness and nausea. Typically these side effects do not require any treatments.

- *Allergic reactions:* The most common allergic reaction symptoms to MRI contrast agents include hives, swelling of the face, rashes, itching, sweating, watery or itchy eyes, and shortness of breath. Frequently, the reactions are mild and can be controlled with medication.

- *Nephrogenic systemic fibrosis:* The most serious side effect caused by MRI contrast is attributed to gadolinium. Patients with renal failure and kidney diseases can't filter the chemical contrast quickly enough and it stays in the body. There it causes a serious medical condition called nephrogenic systemic fibrosis (NSF). NSF symptoms include hardened skin with red patches and are most commonly found in the limbs. Other frequent symptoms include muscle tightening, joint pain, yellow spots on the eyes, and renal and kidney failure. This rare illness has no cure, but can only affect patients with existing kidney problems injected with gadolinium.

Oral Contrast Agents

In MRI oral contrast can be used for enhancement of the gastrointestinal tract. Gadolinium, manganese chelates and iron salts are used for T1 signal enhancement. SPIO, barium sulfate, air and clay have been used to lower T2 signal. Blueberry and green tea having high manganese concentration can also be used for T1 increasing contrast enhancement.

Perflubron, a type of perfluorocarbon, has been used as a gastrointestinal MRI contrast agent for pediatric imaging.

This contrast agent works by reducing the amount of protons in a body cavity. Gadolinium initially disperses through the vascular system and then diffuses into the extracellular space, before moving into the intracellular space. Whilst still circulating within the vessels, magnetic resonance angiography (MRA) can be performed. Gadolinium does not cross the intact blood-brain barrier but helps identifying intracranial lesions with interruption of the barrier, like infection and tumors. It helps to discriminate tumors from edema, low-grade from high-grade tumors, scar tissue from a tumor tissue.

Oral gadolinium is used to highlight loops of bowel to distinguish from surrounding soft tissue. Superparamagnetic agents are more specific hepatic agent and are specially taken up by the Kupffer cells in the liver and help make a distinction between normal liver and malignant tissue.

ULTRASOUND CONTRAST

Ultrasound contrast agents comprise of gas-filled microbubbles measuring less than ten microns. These are also called as 'Echo Enhancing Agents'. They are administered intravenously. Microbubbles have a high degree of echogenicity, and ability to reflect the ultrasound waves. The echogenicity difference between the gas in the microbubbles and the soft tissue surroundings is immense. Thereby, microbubble contrast agents enhance the ultrasound reflections to produce a high echogenicity difference image. Contrast-enhanced ultrasound can be used to image blood perfusion in organs and measure blood flow rate in the heart and other organs.

Ultrasound contrast agents are injected intravenously into the systemic circulation in a small bolus. The microbubbles remain in the systemic circulation

for a certain period of time. During that time, ultrasound waves are directed on the area of interest. The microbubbles reflect unique echo that stands out in contrast to the surrounding tissue. The ultrasound system converts the strong echogenicity into a contrast enhanced image of the area of interest. Similarly the bloodstream's echo is enhanced, thus allow distinguish blood from surrounding tissues.

Ultrasound imaging allows real-time evaluation of blood flow. Since microbubbles can generate such strong signals, a lower intravenous dosage is needed in micrograms. However, microbubbles do not last very long in circulation. They have low circulation time.

The gas inside the shell is generally perfluorocarbons, which are liquids at room temperature but gas at body temperature. The large molecules of perfluorocarbons have slow diffusion and solubility which increase the enhancement time of the contrast medium as compared to air. They are less than 5 microns in size. This is important because they must filter out through the smallest capillary particularly small enough to pass through the pulmonary circulation and the cardiac chambers without disruption. They are stable enough to persist during the examination. 100% of the gas is eliminated from the body through the lungs during normal breathing in about 15 minutes. It circulates only in the vascular spaces and does not enter the tissues. These microbubles enhance the blood in the area of interest and demonstrate the pathology. The component of the shell are absorbed by the blood and later metabolized by the liver.

Ultrasound Contrast Agents in Hepatic Imaging

Some microbubble contrast media have a specific hepatosplenic parenchymal phase. They accumulate in normal hepatic tissue; some are phagocytosed by Kupffer cells in the reticuloendothelial system and others may stay in the sinusoids. The hepatic parenchymal phase, which may last from less than an hour to several days, depending on the specific contrast medium used, may be imaged by bubble-specific modes such as stimulated acoustic emission or pulse inversion imaging. The various gas microbubble contrast media are generally safe with low toxicity in humans.

The need for USG contrast arises when the lesions are isoechoic to the background parenchyma or are diffusely isoechoic and are difficult to pick up or be characterized by B mode ultrasound. Therefore the use of USG contrast has significantly changed the capability of ultrasound imaging. A 38-years-old male reported general weakness was subjected to ultrasound followed by contrast enhanced scan with Sonovue by Bracco (Figs 15.1 A to E).

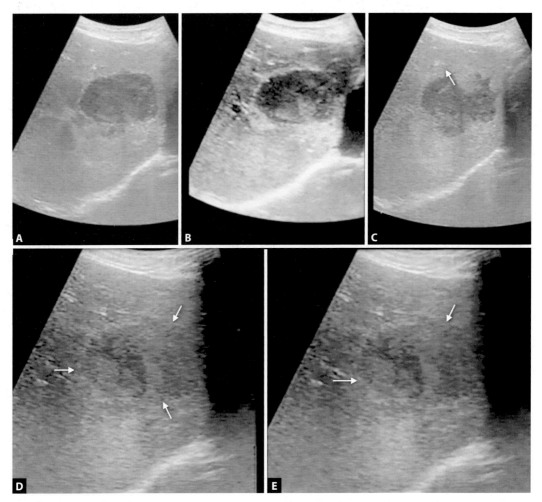

Figs 15.1A to E (A) On ultrasound, right lobe of liver shows a well defined hyoechoic lesion; (B) Intravenous contrast injected, in arterial phase shows outlining the edges of the lesion seen as increased echogenicity of the margins of the lesion; (C) Gradually the circulating contrast shows early filling up the lesion more in the anterior aspect. As a result of peripheral filling there is some change in shape and outline of the lesion; (D and E) Show excellent filling of the lesion resulting in echogenicity isodense to the hepatic tissue which was hyoechoic in precontrast image (A)

Various hepatic ultrasound contrast media available are:

- *Sonavist:* An ultrasound contrast medium consisting of air microbubbles stabilized with a shell of cyanoacrylate. This intravascular contrast medium also has a liver-specific phase, accumulating in the reticuloendothelial system of normal liver tissue.
- *Sonazoid:* An ultrasound contrast medium consisting of perfluorocarbon microbubbles stabilized with surfactants. This intravascular contrast medium also has a liver-specific phase, accumulating in the reticuloendothelial system of normal liver tissue.
- *Levovist:* A second generation ultrasound contrast medium consisting of air microbubbles stabilized

with a shell of palmitic acid. This intravascular contrast medium also has a liver-specific phase, accumulating in normal liver tissue, probably in the sinusoids.

Side-effects

Microbubble contrast agent's side-effects are predominantly minor in nature (headache, nausea). Generalized allergy-like reactions occur rarely. There is the possibility of bioeffects arising from the use of microbubble agents; microvascular rupture can occur where gas bodies are insonated. This may be problematic in areas of sensitivity such as the retina and the brain when imaged through the open fontanelle.

16

Artifacts

Hariqbal Singh

Artifacts are features appearing in reconstructed images which are not present in the true anatomy or original object. These artifacts may mislead to diagnostic quality or may be confused with pathology.

ARTIFACTS IN CONVENTIONAL RADIOGRAPHY

- *Fog:* Film fog is generalized darkening of film. The causes of film fogging are exposure to light, exposure to X-rays or radionuclides, chemical and aging.
  - *Exposure to light:* This occurs when darkroom is not light proof, incorrect safelight bulb, long exposure to safelight.
  - *Exposure to X-rays or radionuclides:* Accidental exposure to X-ray cause film fog. Films should be shielded properly from source of radiation.
  - *Chemical fog:* It occurs due wrong developing techniques.
  - *Age fog:* Either mottled or uniform fogging due to expired shelf life of films.
- *Stain:* Various types of discoloration can appear on films. It can be avoided by use of fresh solutions and proper processing. The discoloration can be
  - *Brown:* When the developer is oxidized it gives brown stain.
  - *Grayish yellow:* When exhausted fixer is used or there is excessive fixation it gives grayish yellow stain.
  - *Grayish white scum:* Incomplete washing causes grayish white scum.
  - *Variegated pattern:* Inadequate rinsing causes different color pattern.
  - *Hyporetention:* Hyporetention is the yellowish stain that appears on finished radiograph due to inadequate washing. Yellowish stain is due to remaining thiosulfate from fixer solution.
- *Marks and defects:* There are various types of markings when films are not handled properly.
  - *Static mark:* Static marks are lightning or tree like black mark on film caused due to friction between film and other objects.

- *Crinkle mark:* They are crescent shaped black or white lines caused due to acute bending of film.
- *Water mark:* Round dark spots are caused on film by water droplets because of migration of silver particles.
- *Cassette marks:* They are caused by foreign matters which leave corresponding marks.
- *Streak:* They usually result from failure to agitate film in developer or fixer, failure to rinse film, failure to stir the solution.
- *Finger marks:* Improper handling with hands cause dark finger.
- *Pressure:* Black and focal artifact caused due improper handling of film.
- *Pi-lines:* Artifact caused on radiograph resulting from dirt or chemical stains on a processing roller in the automatic developer tank. They occur at intervals of pi (3.14) times the diameter of the roller. These are thin, black lines running longitudinally across the X-ray film.
- *Guide shoe mark* are radiographic image artifacts caused by pressure of the guide shoes (the curved metal lips that guide X-ray film in automatic developing systems). These guide shoes leave scratches called ridge lines in the image.
- *Others*
  - *Distorted images:* Improper alignment of the tube, object or film causes distorted image.
  - *Blurred images:* From movement of the patient, film, or tube during exposure.
  - *Double exposure:* Same film is exposed twice.

COMPUTED RADIOGRAPHY ARTIFACTS

Image Acquisition Artifacts (Operator Artifacts)

- *Twin artifacts (double exposure):* If the radiographer accidentally takes two subsequent exposures, it will lead to duplication of images.

Double exposures can lead to errors in interpreting the position of line and catheters.

- *Delayed scanning:* If the phosphor over imaging plate remains unstimulated, it returns to its normal state after a prolonged delay through spontaneous phosphorescence. Thus, a delay between acquisition and processing of the image will lead to fading of the image.
- *Uncollimated images:* If the image collimation is not parallel to the imaging plate, proper borders will not be recognized, resulting in bizarre or nondiagnostic images.
- *Exposure through the back of the cassette:* Any exposure through the back of the cassette will leave its own pattern of artifacts.
- *Improper grid usage Moiré pattern:* Grids with low grid line rates are known to cause a Moiré pattern, resulting in suboptimal image quality.
- *Care and carelessness:* CR cassettes with imaging plates must be stored and handled carefully. Buckling occurs as a result of mishandling of imaging plates by radiographers during the cleaning process, which causes kink.
- *Light bulb effect:* Artifactual darkening of the lower and outer portions of an image relative to the remainder of the image is caused by back-scattered radiation entering the photo stimulable phosphor (PSP) imaging plate from the patient's bed. The source of this artifact can be attributed to an increased exposure for obese patients or uncollimated X-ray beam. Reducing backscatter by lowering the kilovoltage or by more precise collimation will limit the prevalence and impact of this artifact.

Image Processing Artifact

Image-processing artifacts can arise from the imaging plate, the rollers in the CR reader that carry the imaging plate, and the plate reader, in which a laser is used to scan the imaging plate.

- *Imaging plate artifact:* Imaging plate artifacts arise due to cracks resulting from aging of the imaging plate and roller-induced artifacts. As the imaging plate passes through the plate reader, the imaging plate bends over the rollers. Over a period of time, the plates show signs of mechanical stress in the form of cracks. These cracks are usually first visible on the edges of the imaging plate. As the deterioration progresses, cracks appear closer to the central imaging plate area. In some cases, artifacts are the result of dust particles on the imaging plate.
- *Roller artifact:* Disparity artifacts are due to malfunctioning of rollers in the digitizer, which causes defective scanning. The defective scanning alters the image contrast in the upper and lower half of the images. Focal radiopacities, which appear as dots, are caused by mechanical damage of the imaging plate during its transport through the rollers. Dust on the rubber rollers is another source of artifacts. Artifacts can be caused by slipping of the feed rollers, resulting in images being half read. Periodic cleaning and recalibration of the feed rollers is of immense importance to prevent slippage of the feed rollers. The light collection guide also needs to be cleaned, but only by authorized service personnel of the manufacturer.
- *Plate reader artifact:* Dirt over the light guide is seen as a linear radiodense line on radiograph. The light guide inside the scan unit should be cleaned by the manufacturer's service personnel.
- *Cassette-related artifacts:* Scatter radiation through the back of the cassette produces black lines. These lines are analogous to the place where the lead coating was cracked or weakened.
- *Improper erasure setting:* Before inserting the cassette into the digitizer, the body part should be selected properly, because this setting determines the right erasure cycle time for the body part. If either the body part is erroneously selected or the power of the erasure halogen lamp is weakened, a residual image is left on the imaging plate. This is confirmed by another exposure on the same imaging plate, where an image resulting from the previous exposure overlaps the new image.

ULTRASOUND AND DOPPLER ARTIFACTS

- *Acoustic shadowing:* Acoustic shadowing can be created through diffraction and refraction on intersections edge. The acoustic shadowing artifact is the loss of information below a dense object as the majority of the sound energy is reflected back by the object. Bone, air, foreign bodies and calcification stop the transmission of sound waves producing a 'sonic shadow' which is a dark region distal to the echogenic obstructing region. Comet tail artifact is part of this.
- *Aliasing artifact:* Echoes of deep lying structures within the body do not always come from the latest emitted sound pulse and can produce an aliasing artifact. This artifact can be problematical at Spectral or Color Doppler examinations. Aliasing of the data displayed in pulsed wave technology is utilized as a benefit in determining transitions from laminar to turbulent flow.
- *Beam width artifact:* When the ultrasound beam is wider than the diameter of the lesion being

scanned, normal tissues which lie immediately adjacent to the lesion are included within the beam width, and their echotexture is averaged in with that of the lesion. Thus, what appears to be the echogenicity of the lesion is really that of the lesion plus the averaged normal tissues.

- *Cross talk artifact:* Cross talk is an ultrasound artifact in which strong sound signals in one directional channel leak into another, appearing as a mirror image of the spectral display on the opposite side of the baseline. Cross talk distinguishes the condition of undesired crossover of transmitted sound waves into the receiving transducer in a continuous wave Doppler system.

- *Duplication artifact:* Duplication artifacts is created through diffraction and refraction on interfaces, also if the acoustical impedances of tissue is too much different and the ultrasound is reflected multiple on tissue layers, where the detected echo does not come from the shortest sound path.

- *Enhancement artifact:* The enhancement artifact appears as a hyperechoic signal. The attenuation of the ultrasound wave in fluids is much lower as the attenuation in other tissues; therefore tissues distal to fluid are enhanced.

- *Mirror artifact:* Mirror image artifacts (mirroring) can occur if the acoustical impedances of the tissue is too much different and the ultrasound is reflected multiple times on tissue layers. The echo detected does not come from the shortest sound path; the sound is reflected off an angle to another interface so that like a real mirror, the artifact shows up as the virtual object. The angle of reflection is equal to the angle of incidence.

- *Rayleigh scattering:* Rayleigh scattering is the back scattering of ultrasound from blood. The echoes detected from blood are created through interference between scattered wavelets from numerous point scatterers. The intensity of the backscattered echoes is proportional to the total number of scatterers, which means that the echo amplitude is proportional to the square root of the total number of scatterers.

- *Refraction artifact:* Different sound velocities in tissue are causing refraction artifacts. With convex lens transducers, sound beam refraction at the skin interface can alter the transducer's focusing characteristics and beam profile, cause element to element nonuniformity, and cause phase changes in the acoustic wave. These cumulative refraction induced errors degrade the image quality through distortion and loss of resolution.

- *Reverbation artifact:* Reverberation artifacts are produced from the multiple reflections from an object if the acoustical impedances of tissue layers are too much different and the detected echo does not run the shortest sound path because it bounces back and forth between the object and the transducer. In a reverberation artifact, the sound wave is reflected back into the body from the transducer-skin interface.

- *Grating lobe or side lobe artifact:* The dimension of the ultrasound beam and the transducer array are the origin of grating-lobe artifacts (also called side lobe artifact). Grating lobes as side lobes are off-axis secondary ultrasound beams projecting at predictable angles to the main lobe. Side lobes are too small to produce important artifacts.

COMPUTED TOMOGRAPHY ARTIFACTS

Computed tomography is more prone to artifacts than conventional radiographs because the image is reconstructed from million independent detectors. The types of artifact that can occur are:

- *Streaking:* Due to an inconsistency in a single detector measurement.

- *Shading:* Due to a group of channels or views deviating gradually from the true measurement.

- *Rings:* Due to errors in an individual detector calibration.

- *Distortion:* Due to helical reconstruction.

- *Physics based artifacts:* Resulting from the physical processes involved in the acquisition of CT data
  - *Beam hardening:* As the X-ray beam passes through an object, it becomes harder, i.e. its mean energy increases, because the lower energy photons are absorbed more rapidly than the higher energy photons. Two types:
    - ◆ *Cupping artifacts:* X-rays passing through the middle portion of a uniform cylindrical phantom are hardened more than those passing though the edges because they are passing through more material. The harder it becomes, the less the beam is attenuated, so when it reaches the detectors it gives a higher signal than would be expected if it had not been hardened. The resultant attenuation profile therefore differs from the ideal profile that would be obtained if there were no beam hardening.
    - ◆ *Streaks and dark bands:* In very heterogeneous cross sections, dark bands or streaks can appear between two dense objects in an image. They occur because the portion of the beam that passes through one of the objects at certain tube positions is hardened less than when it passes through both objects at other tube positions. Built-in features for minimizing beam hardening.

Filtration: A piece of attenuating material will filter out the lower energy components before it passes through the patient.

Calibration corrections: Some manufacturers provide phantoms which allow the detectors to be calibrated with compensation tailored for the beam hardening effects.

Beam hardening correction software: An iterative correction algorithm may be automatically applied when images of bony regions are being reconstructed. This helps minimize blurring of the bone/soft tissue interface in brain scans and also reduces the appearance of dark bands in nonhomogeneous cross sections.

Avoidance of beam hardening by the operator is sometimes possible to avoid scanning bony regions, either by means of patient positioning or by tilting the gantry.

- *Partial volume:* Partial volume cause shading artifacts when the dense objects lie off-center by underestimation of CT number for dense objects. Partial volume artifacts can be expected in images of any part of the body where the anatomy is changing rapidly in the z direction, for example in the posterior fossa. They can best be avoided by using a thin acquisition slice. To reduce image noise, thicker slices can be reconstructed from the acquired data.

- *Under sampling:* Too coarse a sampling interval leads to misregistration by the computer of information relating to sharp edges and small objects. This leads to an effect known as aliasing, where fine striations appear in the image.

  Using high resolution techniques such as quarter-detector shift or flying focal spot.

- *Photon starvation:* A potential source of serious streaking artifacts is photon starvation, which can occur in highly attenuating areas such as the shoulders. When the beam passes horizontally through the widest part of the patient, insufficient photons reach the detectors and very noisy projections are produced. The noise is magnified when the views are reconstructed, resulting in horizontal streaks in the image.

  It can be minimized by automatic tube current modulation which varies the tube current during the course of each rotation. This allows sufficient photons to pass through the widest parts of the patient without unnecessary dose to the narrower parts.

  Adaptive filtration: A type of adaptive filtration is used which smoothes each projection only in areas of low signal.

- *Patient based artifacts:* Caused by such factors as patient movement or the presence of metallic materials in or on the patient

  - *Metallic materials:* The presence of metal objects in the scan field can lead to severe streaking artifacts. They occur because the density of the metal is beyond the normal range that can be handled by the computer.

    Avoidance of metal artifacts by the operator by asking the patients to take off removable metal objects for nonremovable items, such as dental fillings, prosthetic devices and surgical clips, it is sometimes possible to use gantry angulations to exclude the metal inserts from scans of nearby anatomy.

  - *Patient motion:* Patient motion can cause misregistration artifacts, which appear as shading in the reconstructed image. Steps can be taken to prevent voluntary motion, but some involuntary motion may be unavoidable during body scanning.

    The use of positioning aids is sufficient to prevent voluntary movement in the majority of patients. In some cases, e.g. pediatrics, however, it is necessary to immobilize the patient by means of sedation. Using as short a scan time as possible helps minimize artifacts. Respiratory motion can be prevented if the patient is able to hold their breath for the duration of the scan.

    Some scanner models use over scan for axial body scans, whereby an extra 10% or so is added to the standard 360° rotation. The repeated projections are averaged, which helps reduce motion artifacts.

- *Scanner based artifacts:* Result from imperfections in scanner function

  - *Ring artifacts:* If one of the detectors is out of calibration, it will give a consistently erroneous reading at each angular position, resulting in a circular artifact. The presence of circular artifacts in an image is an indication that the detector gain needs recalibration.

- *Helical and multislice artifact:* Dependent on the image reconstruction method employed

  - *Helical artifacts in the transverse plane:* The artifacts are a result of rapidly changing structures in the z-direction. If a helical scan is performed of a cone-shaped phantom lying along the z-axis of the scanner, the resultant trans axial images should appear circular. In fact, however, their shape is distorted because of the weighting function used in the helical interpolation algorithm. For some projection angles, the image is influenced more by contributions from wider parts of the cone in front of the scan plane and for other projection angles, contributions from narrower parts of the cone behind the scan plane predominate. Minimization of helical artifacts is by using a pitch of 1 rather than a higher pitch where possible, a 180° rather than a 360° helical interpolator and thin acquisition slice rather than thick.

- *Helical artifacts in multislice scanning:* Multi-slice scanners are prone to a similar type of trans axial image distortion due to helical interpolation as single-slice scanners. Their severity is reduced by the use of a z-filter helical interpolator instead of a two point interpolator.

- *Multiplanar and 3D reconstructions:*
    - ♦ *Stair step artifacts:* Stair step artifacts appear around the edges of structures in multiplanar and 3D reconstructions when wide collimations and nonoverlapping reconstruction intervals are used. They are less severe with helical scanning, which permits reconstruction of overlapping slices without the extra dose to the patient that occurs when overlapping axial scans are performed. Stair-step artifacts are virtually eliminated in multiplanar and 3D reconstructions of thin slice data from today's multi-slice scanners.
    - ♦ *Zebra artifacts:* Faint stripes may be apparent because the helical interpolation process gives rise to a degree of noise in homogeneity along the z-axis. This 'zebra' effect becomes more pronounced away from the axis of rotation because the noise inhomogeneity is worse off-axis.

- *Cone beam effect:* As the tube and detectors rotate around the patient, the data collected by each detector corresponds to a volume contained between two cones, instead of the ideal flat plane. Artifacts are more pronounced for the outer detector rows than for the inner ones, where the data collected corresponds more closely to a plane. They occur around off-axis objects.

Manufacturers' techniques for minimizing cone beam artifacts.

They can be minimized by various forms of cone beam reconstruction are used.

MAGNETIC RESONANCE IMAGING ARTIFACTS

Artifacts are imaging findings that are not actual part the original image or what the image should have been.

It is important to recognize them, so that misdiagnosis can be avoided as they can sufficiently degrade images to cause a misdiagnosis; it can obscure pathology or create a false one. Sources of such artifacts can be broadly divided into

- Movement related artifacts
- Non motional artifacts.

Movement related artifacts can be again divided into:

- *Gross body movement related artifacts:* MRI is motion sensitive as the images are based on timing sequences; these cause artifacts to appear in reconstructed images. Movement can occur during RF pulses, between RF pulses, during data sampling and between phase—encoding sequences. Gross body movement in the patient may occur in all three dimensions but the artifacts propagate in the two dimensional phase—encoding dimension (Fig. 16.1). Random patient movement, gastro-intestinal peristalsis or eye ball movements may cause such artifacts. When motion is periodic occurring in a cyclical pattern it results in complete or incomplete replication of the affected vowels, commonly referred to as "Ghosting".

- *Physiological motion related artifacts:* These can be caused by respiratory motion artifacts, cardiac motion artifacts; fluid tissue pulsation artifacts (blood flow, CSF flow). The ghosting artifact can arise from respiration due to high signal intensity of fat which moves with breathing. These artifacts can be minimized using techniques such as: breath holds technique, respiratory gating, respiratory ordered phase encoding (ROPE), and navigator gating, fat suppression sequences such as STIR sequences. Abdominal movement during respiration can be suppressed by using a compression belt across the abdomen.

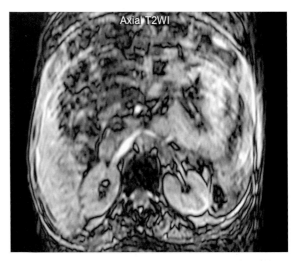

Fig. 16.1 Axial T2WI shows motion blurring of the image with image distortion due to respiratory motion

In cardiac MRI, continuous contraction and dilatation of the cardiac chambers constitute a physiological motion resulting in blurring of cardiac structures. To eliminate such artifacts cardiac gating technique is used, the imaging sequence is triggered by the R-wave and the data is collected during the same period of the cardiac cycle for each TR period.

Fluid pulsation artifacts due to pulsatile CSF flow may show on MRI as areas of signal void and also as ghosting in phase—encoding direction. Gradient movement rephrasing (GMR) is a method of balancing the phase for both stationary and moving nuclear spins. This technique has been successful in eliminating CSF pulsatile flow artifacts in gradient echo images of head and spine.

Fluid pulsation artifacts due to blood flow may produce a range of artifacts:
- Pulsatile blood flow may produce ghost artifacts in the phase—encoding direction
- Flowing blood can cause an anomalously low or high signal intensity.
- Flow signal can be mismapped on the image and appear outside the vessel in the frequency encoding direction.

Techniques such as cardiac (peripheral) gating, swapping phase frequency encoding axes, presaturation pulses are useful to eliminate artifacts due to blood flow. Presaturation bands are used in spin echo imaging of the head and whole body, since venous and arterial blood flow occur in opposite directions, "presaturation slabs" are applied on either side of the imaging volume to saturate flow in either direction, this principle is important in MR angiography.

Non-motional artifacts: These can be broadly divided into:
- Patient related artifacts
- MRI scanner related artifacts.

Patient-related Artifacts

- *Extrinsic type:* Ferromagnetic metal artifacts show up as characteristic geometric distortion with a region of near zero signal intensity adjacent to a bright region Removal of the metal object eliminates this type of artifact.
- Magnetic susceptibility is tendency of material to become magnetized when placed in magnetic field. Caused by material with large differences in susceptibility create local disturbance in magnetic field resulting in non linear changes of resonant frequency, which in turn creates image distortion and signal changes leading to signal void in image. (Figs 16.2A to D).

- *Intrinsic type (magnetic susceptibility):* Diamagnetic effects are apparent at anatomical interfaces like between adjacent tissues depending on their degree of polarization with respect to the magnetic field applied. Tissues such as cortical bone or air filled cavities have little polarisable hydrogen atoms whereas soft tissues have hydrogen atoms in greater numbers available to get polarized by the magnetic field. The patient may also disturb the magnetic field because of increase in concentration of hemoglobin that may occur following bleeding, as concentrated hemoglobin is ferromagnetic due to its high iron content. Spin echo sequences minimize these types of artifacts. Chemical shift artifacts arise from the frequency difference between the hydrogen nuclei in water and the hydrogen nuclei in fat and tissues when subjected to the magnetic field. This frequency difference is defined as chemical shift in MR spectroscopy, is usually expressed as a fraction of the Larmor frequency. Thus two static artifacts can be generated by chemical shift—signal misrepresentation and phase cancellation. Chemical shift artifacts can be minimized by performing imaging at low magnetic field strengths, by also increasing the frequency bandwidth or by decreasing the field of view (FOV).

MRI Scanner-related Artifacts

- *Gibbs phenomenon (ringing artifact) or truncation artifact:* This is caused by the under-sampling of high spatial frequencies at sharp boundaries in the image. Lack of appropriate high-frequency components leads to an oscillation at a sharp transition known as a ringing artifact. The artifact occurs near the sharp boundaries, where high contrast transitions in the object occur. It appears as multiple, regularly spaced parallel ripples of alternating bright and dark signal parallel to tissue interface (Figs 16.3A to C). This artifact can be eliminated by increasing the phase-encodings or reduce the FOV.
- *Aliasing or wrap around artifact* occurs when the FOV is smaller than the area to be scanned. The region to be scanned lies outside the FOV but within the slice volume. The region outside the FOV is seen wrapped around on the opposite side. It can be caused by under sampling of the frequencies contained within the return signal. This can be generally seen in the end slices of the 3D acquisition (Fig. 16.3D). It can be corrected by increasing the FOV, but it decreases resolution. It can be also reduced by oversampling the data in the frequency direction (standard) and increasing

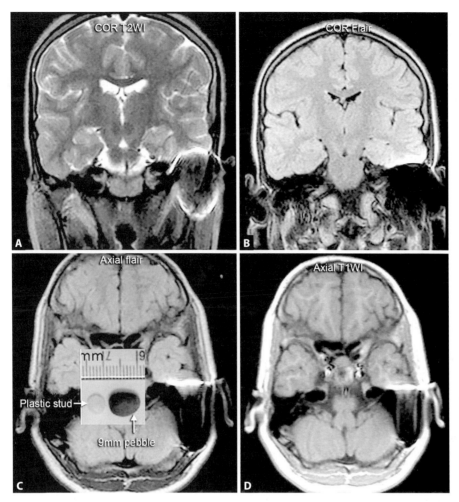

Figs 16.2A to D Axial T1WI shows image distortion with signal void in the region of the petrous portion of left temporal bone due to susceptibility artifact in a fifteen year old female patient with history of recurrent episodes headache, giddiness and loss of consciousness over last three years. Small pebble and a plastic stud as foreign body was found and removed from the left external auditory canal (inset). Scan was repeated and magnetic susceptibility artifact disappeared

phase steps in the phase-encoded direction—phase compensation (time or SNR penalty). Surface coil can be used so no signal is detected outside of FOV.

- *Zebra* artifacts or bands occur due to instabilities of magnetic field gradients due to overheated or overloaded gradient coils, they can produce loss of spatial resolution or even image ghosting in the phase—encoding direction. Eddy current compensation and active shielding of gradient coils are needed to prevent such artifacts.

- *Noise* artifacts occur when radiofrequencies from sources like television, radio interfere with the MRI scanner RF signal. It can produce graininess to the MR images. In such situations RF distortion will be seen in images. To counter this problem a RF shielding cage (Faraday cage) is constructed around the MRI scan room. The shielding material often used is copper or aluminum grids.

- *Zipper* artifacts can occur due to RF surface coils placed close to the patient. Artifacts appear as "image shading" or in worst cases as "linear serrated images" resembling a zipper (Fig. 16.3E). Adjusting the RF surface coil and selecting a smaller FOV helps to minimize this artifact.

- *Center line* artifacts, here the artifact appear in the center in frequency encoding direction or parallel to the phase encoding direction. It occurs due to RF interference as the RF transmitter and receiver are placed close together. This type of artifacts can be eliminated by alternating the phase of the RF pulse and by isolating the receiver amplifier chain.

- *Shading* artifacts are seen as foci of relatively reduced signal intensity involving some part of

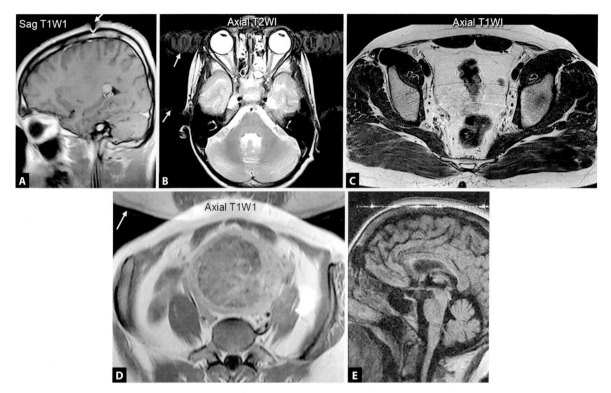

Figs 16.3A to E Sagittal T1WI (A) shows susceptibility artifact over the scalp due to coupling gel. Patient had come for MRI after EEG examination. Multiple, regularly spaced parallel bands of alternating bright and dark signal seen parallel to the orbit and the petrous portion of the temporal bones (B) is referred as Gibbs artifact. Similar parallel bands are seen in pelvis (C). Axial T1WI shows (D) overlapping wrap around of the posterior abdominal wall over the anterior. It is called wrap around artifact. Linear serrated images (E) resembling a zipper are seen and is referred as zipper artifact

the MR image. Some causes for this type of artifact are magnetic field inhomogeneity, partial volume averaging. Malfunction of the RF transmitter, amplifier or receiver and excessive absorption of power can all lead to shading artifacts. Reducing the slice thickness and scanning in two planes (transversely and sagittally) helps to eliminate shading artifacts.

- *Crosstalk* most MRI scans are acquired as multiple two dimensional slices. From one slice to the next only the RF frequency is changed. So, if the slices are placed too closely, the tail of one RF slice excitation can partially excite the neighboring slice. This effect can be minimized by interleaving the slice acquisitions, so that within this time the magnetization of the adjacent slice will recover towards equilibrium value so that only the slice that is excited by the RF gives the signals back to the receiver.

Partial volume averaging: Although the MR image appears to be two dimensional, all the information within the slice is averaged and contributes to the final image. For instance a tumor that is only partially contained within a slice will appear to be different from the one that spans the slice. This phenomenon is called partial volume averaging and it gives the radiologist an incomplete picture of the lesion. Thus to avoid missing the lesion due to this phenomenon it is necessary to image the region of interest in more than one orientation (sagittal, coronal, axial sections).

17
Computed Radiography and Digital Radiography

Shrikant Nagare

The advances in the medical imaging field has been considerably impacted in recent years by the emergence of digital imaging modalities, including computed radiography and digital radiography, also known as direct digital radiography. Digital systems allow for a greater flexibility in radiology workload.

Conventional radiography involves use of intensifying screens to form the latent image on a radiographic film which is further chemically process to acquire the analog image. Acceptable film quality is possible within a narrow exposure limits. Limited exposure latitude results in frequent under and overexposure of films. The conventional radiography is time and labor intensive hence inefficient. Limitations of conventional processing includes processing related artifacts, fixed image contrast and density, limited magnification, film quality deterioration with time and incompatibility with electronic imaging.

In digital radiography system a digital detector replaces the screens. The two basic types of digital radiography systems are computed radiography system (CR) and direct digital radiography system (DR).

COMPUTED RADIOGRAPHY

Computed radiography system uses a photostimulable phosphor (PSP) plate enclosed in light tight cassette (Fig. 17.1). PSP plate replaces film and screen in film screen radiography. PSP plate is coated with europium-activated barium fluorohalide (BaFX:Eu). Halide used is either a bromide, iodide or a combination of both. As the plate is exposed to X-rays, the information is captured in the form of trapped electrons. The captured image is acquired by exposing the image plate in CR reader. The imaging plate is scanned by a red laser beam. This laser beam excites the trapped electrons leading to ejection of electrons from higher

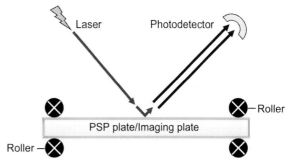

Fig. 17.1 Schematic mechanism of CR system: Imaging plate coated with photostimulable phosphor (PSP) exposed to X-rays and contains image data. In CR reader imaging plate is read using red laser beam, which is swept across the plate by a rotating polygonal mirror. The light emitted by imaging plate is converted into electrical signal and used to form image

energy state to lower energy state. During this process they emit energy in the form of blue light which is captured by a light guide and converted into electrical signals. The electrical signal is amplified, digitized and used to form the image. The imaging PSP plate can be reused after exposed to white light. Patient information and cassette ID is linked to CR reader using a bar code embedded in PSP plate.

The acquired image can be post processed for windowing, edge and contrast enhancement. Multiple exact copies of the post processed images can be made. The digital image can be displayed on multiple working stations for reporting and viewing. This digital image can be used for the teleradiology and computer aided diagnosis (CAD). Picture archiving and communication system (PACS) allows archiving and retrieval of the digital image and helps in developing a filmless and pollution free, environment friendly department. Existing multiple X-ray equipment can be used to expose cassettes which can be read by a single CR system.

DIRECT DIGITAL RADIOGRAPHY

Digital radiography (DR) system uses a flat panel detector to acquire latent image which is transferred directly to a review monitor without need for a cassettes and readers. DR plates are used with mobile X-ray units or in bucky trays using wireless remote technology to transfer the image data. The similarities between CR and DR technology are primarily in the digital format of the resultant image. Both CR and DR image formats are compatible for storage in a digital picture archiving communication system and the appearance of the digital images can be manipulated.

Four different types of DR systems are available depending upon the type of detectors used in them.

1. *Flat panel detector (FPD) based systems:* Thin film transistor (TFT) arrays made up of amorphous silicon are used in the formation of FPD. The FPD assembly consists of an X-ray converter, which is either photo scintillator or photoconductor layered on a TFT matrix on a glass substrate. Each TFT element has a capacitor and a switching transistor. Gait and drain lines are connected to each transistor and capacitor, enabling active readout of charges from each detector element separately. The flat panel detectors are of two types depending on the method and material used for the conversion of X-rays into electrical signals: (i) Direct X-ray conversion type that uses a photoconductor and (ii) Indirect X-ray conversion type that uses a photo scintillator/phosphor screen (Fig. 17.2).

    Direct conversion type of detectors use amorphous selenium photoconductor sandwiched between two electrodes to which high voltage is applied. The X-rays are directly converted to electrical signal, when X-rays fall on this layer by producing, electrons and holes. Indirect conversion FPDs first convert X-rays to light in a scintillator/phosphor, which in turn is then detected by photodiodes and TFT arrays. Thallium-doped Cesium Iodide (CsI) is the most commonly used phosphor material. It is structured in the form of thin needle-shaped crystals. Another material used is turbid gadolinium oxysulfide or Gadox (Gd_2O_2S).

2. *2D or area charge couple device (CCD) array-based systems:* In these DR systems the X-rays are absorbed and converted into visible light in large scintillators or phosphors. This light is channeled by means of mirrors/lenses/prisms and fiber optically coupled to a much smaller light-sensitive CCD array. These detectors are relatively bulky, but are less costly than FPDs.

3. *Slot-scanning types:* A narrow fan beam moves across the anatomical region along with two precisely aligned moving slit collimators, one on either side of the patient, are used in such systems. This prevents scatter radiation from reaching the detector. It works somewhat like a scanogram in CT.

4. *Photon counting type DR system:* Photon counting type of DR system has construction similar to the slot scanning type but uses a different type of detector. These systems use a multislit detector made of crystalline Silicon (Si) as a scintillator. Absorbed X-rays produce electrons and holes. Each of these events is counted in a meter with time corresponding to the spatial location along the direction of X-ray fan beam sweep. Each absorbed X-ray photon results in a unit count regardless of the photon energy.

CR and DR have many similarities. Both use a medium to capture X-ray energy and both produce

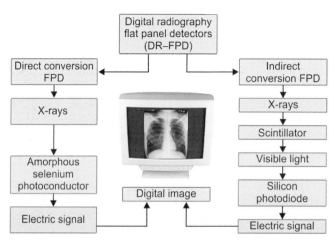

Fig. 17.2 Types of DR flat panel detectors (i) Direct conversion flat panel detectors: X-rays are converted to electric signal by amorphous selenium photoconductor; (ii) Indirect conversion flat panel detector: X-rays are converted to visible light by Scintillator, which is further converted to electric signal by silicon photodiode. Electric signal is converted to digital image by TFT arrays

Table 17.1 Comparison of computed radiography and digital radiography

	Computed radiography	Digital radiography
Steps required	Loading of cassette in bucky	No need to load cassette in bucky
	Positioning of patient for exposure	Positioning of patient for exposure
	Positioning of X-ray tube	Positioning of X-ray tube
	Performing X-ray exposure	Performing X-ray exposure
	Transport of exposed cassette to CR reader	Image captured by digital detectors is transferred to the viewing station via LAN (Local Area Network) connection automatically (No cassettes required)
	IP bar code reading and loading cassette in CR reader	
	Assess image quality	Assess image quality
Image acquisition process	A photostimulable plate (PSP) within the cassette is exposed to a X-ray beam	Built-in image capture plates are used no cassettes required
	Latent image is captured in the plate as electrons in the phosphor are excited when exposed to radiation	Large-area, flat-panel detectors with integrated TFT readout mechanisms, integrated PSP plate scanning mechanisms, or optic lens used to translate the analog image to a digital image
	Exposed cassette is placed in a reader to capture and analyze the image data	
	Laser and analog-to-digital converter translates signal to digital binary code	
Image quality	Digital environment presents opportunities to improve image interpretation	Digital environment presents opportunities to improve image interpretation
	Potential for lower image noise and lower radiation exposure	Potential for lower image noise and lower radiation exposure
		Offer potential for better image quality with lower radiation dose than CR
Potential advantages and disadvantages	Unlimited manipulation and positioning of the image receptor for cross-table projections is possible	Only few DR systems can perform cross-table lateral and decubitus procedures
	Relatively slower workflow due to loading unloading of X-ray cassettes	Faster workflow due to elimination of cassettes
	PACS/DICOM compatible	PACS/DICOM compatible
	Possibility of repetitive motion injuries to cassettes	No damage to detectors related to motion
	Longer turnaround time for viewing image	Shorter turnaround time for viewing image hence freeing of staff time
	Lower cost as compared to DR	Higher costs
	Previously installed X-ray equipment can be upgraded to CR system	Needs installation of new equipment

a digital image. CR generally involves the use of a cassette that houses the imaging plate, similar to traditional film-screen systems, to record the image whereas DR typically captures the image directly onto a flat panel detector without the use of a cassette. Image processing or enhancement can be applied on DR images as well as CR images due to the digital format of each (Table 17.1).

18

Positron Emission Tomography-Computed Tomography

Sikandar Shaikh

Positron emission tomography (PET) is an imaging modality that identifies the presence of a metabolically active tumor within the body after injecting a radioactive substance.

A CT scan uses X-rays to provide an anatomical image of the patient.

A positron emission tomography-computed tomography machine is a single device that combines both modalities to produce an image that shows the metabolic functional information from the PET image and the anatomical information from the CT scan. The resultant data is displayed as a combined, or fused, PET-CT image (Fig. 18.1).

Normal cells use glucose for their day-to-day function but in general the glucose uptake in most normal cells is relatively low. Active tumors tend to have a much greater metabolic rate than most normal cells and consequently use considerably more glucose.

Cardiac muscle, for example, preferentially uses free fatty acids as an energy source, but it can also use glucose, lipids, or amino acids if required. As a result, the glucose uptake within the heart varies among people and can change considerably within an individual over a short period in relation to the blood glucose. Brain cells do not have the ability to use any fuel other than glucose and consequently the glucose activity within the brain is always high.

TRACERS USED FOR POSITRON EMISSION TOMOGRAPHY

Glucose

Flurodeoxyglucose (FDG) is an analog of glucose that is labeled to the radioactive positron emitter Flourine-18. The FDG is injected intravenously and is taken up by normal and tumor cells alike in a fashion similar to glucose. F is a radioactive substance which emits radioactive particles called positrons. FDG has a half-life of approximately 109 minutes. Other radioisotope-positron emitters which can be used are carbon-11, nitrogen-13 and oxygen-15 having much shorter half life.

Poor Performance of FDG

In lesions like prostate cancer, hepatoma, renal cell-low grade carcinoma, bronchoalveolar carcinoma (occasionally) and mucinous adenocarcinoma low performance of FDG is noted.

Procedure

Patients should arrive fasting for at least four hours. This ensures that most tissues are using free fatty acids as their energy source. Diabetic patients are advised to take their normal insulin or medication. Then the dose of tracer is given intravenously. The patient is advised to lie still for approximately 45 minutes to allow the FDG time to accumulate in metabolically active cells. Any unnecessary patient movement during this uptake period can result in muscular uptake. Patients who are tense during this time often show physiological uptake within the muscles of the neck. The PET-CT scan is normally carried out from the base of skull to mid-thigh level, the so-called whole body scan. Patients with melanoma have a whole body scan from skull vertex to feet. This is because of the widespread and unpredictable lymphatic dissemination that characterizes this disease. Patients with head and neck disease often have scans that include the entire skull, and patients with soft tissue sarcomas may also require additional views. After the CT images are acquired the patient is then scanned for PET.

A semi quantitative method called the *Standardized Uptake Value* (SUV) is often used as parameter for measuring the uptake by the lesion (Table 18.1).

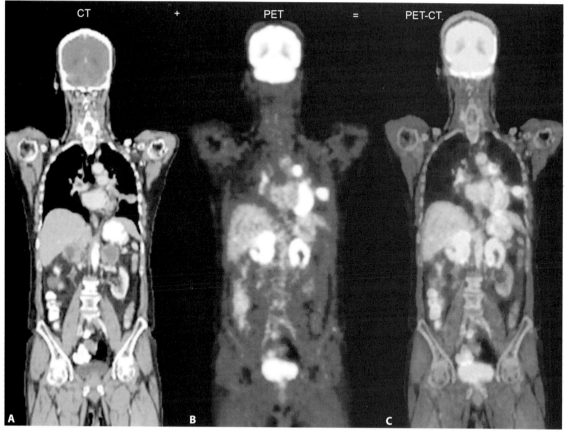

Figs 18.1A to C Coronal reconstructed CT image: (A) of thorax and abdomen showing mass in lung and mass lesion in both adrenals. Post FDG injection PET; (B) and fused PET-CT; (C) image shows increased tracer uptake in lung mass and bilateral adrenals, suggestive of carcinoma lung with adrenal metastases (*For color version, see Plate 3*)

Table 18.1 Standardized uptake value (SUV) for various body tissues

Sr. No.	Region	SUV
1.	Soft tissue	0.6–0.8
2.	Liver	2.2–2.5
3.	Kidneys	3.3–3.5
4.	Neoplasm	5.0–20

LUNG CANCER

PET-CT is useful for assessment of the solitary pulmonary nodule (SPN), staging of nonsmall cell lung cancer (NSCLC) (Figs 18.1A to C), assessment of mediastinal lymphadenopathy, identification of distant metastatic disease, detection of recurrent disease, radiotherapy planning and response to therapy assessment and as a prognostic indicator.

Approximately 85% of metabolically active pulmonary nodules are malignant. If an FDG positive pulmonary nodule is found, it should be assumed to be malignant until proved otherwise.

False positive cases are noted in granulomatous conditions, inflammation, sarcoidosis, infection and adenomas. False negative cases are noted in bronchoalveolar cancer, scar adenocarcinoma, carcinoid tumors and neuroendocrine tumors.

LYMPHOMA

Positron emission tomography-computed tomography is useful to assess response to therapy/residual disease (Figs 18.2A to C), identify recurrent disease, initial diagnosis and staging, identify suitable sites for biopsy, disease surveillance and radiotherapy planning. False-positive cases are seen in infection, cardiac/bowel uptake, thymic hyperplasia and inflammation. False-negative cases are seen in MALT lymphoma, lymphocytic NHL and CML.

COLORECTAL CANCER

The risk factors include age, diet, polyps, chronic ulcerative colitis and familial polyposis coli (FAP). Adenocarcinoma is most common histological type.

Clinical indications for PET-CT in colorectal cancer are assessment of recurrent disease, assessment of

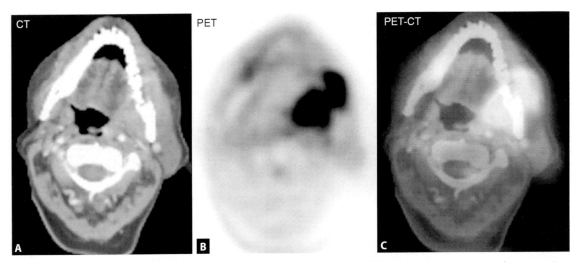

Figs 18.2A to C Operated case of tongue carcinoma, axial CT shows a lesion (A) There is intense tracer uptake suggestive of recurrence of tumor (B, C) (*For color version, see Plate 3*)

tumor response to chemo/radiotherapy, assessment of a mass that is difficult to biopsy and unexplained rising CEA in patients with a history of colorectal cancer and normal conventional imaging.

False-positive cases are noted in physiological uptake, inflammation, polyps, stoma site/postoperative changes. False-negative cases are noted in small bowel disease, mucinous secreting tumors, peritoneal metastases and carcinoid tumors.

HEAD AND NECK CANCERS

Clinical indications for PET-CT are staging primary head and neck cancer, identifying sites of recurrence, distinguishing postoperative change from residual disease, finding the site of an unknown primary tumor, assessing the response to therapy and acting as a prognostic tool.

SKIN CANCER

Positron emission tomography-computed tomography is useful for staging of patients with suspected nodal or distant metastatic involvement, staging of suspicious lesions at presentation, restaging patients prior to surgical metastectomy, confirmation of suspected recurrence and detecting almost all melanoma metastases greater than 1 cm in diameter, in the detection of distant disease. PET-CT avoids unnecessary surgery and results in significant management change. It is best employed in patients with suspected nodal or distant metastatic involvement, or a high risk of such spread.

GYNECOLOGICAL MALIGNANCIES

Ovarian Carcinomas

Ovarian cancer is associated with late presentation and poor prognosis. At present, the role of FDG-PET has largely been in assessment for recurrent disease (Figs 18.3A to C). With PET-CT, the investigation is likely to be even more successful, particularly in reducing the number of false-positive reports.

Carcinoma of the Cervix

Both CT and MR (more often used) are used to stage carcinoma of the cervix. The limitation of this structural staging is often, as is the case for all tumors, the arbitrary 1 cm cut off for differentiation of malignant from benign disease. It is now accepted that small nodes can harbor disease and large nodes may only be reactive. As lymph node staging is fundamental in the management of cervical cancer both in terms of survival and treatment, accurate assessment of nodal involvement is required.

UNKNOWN PRIMARY TUMORS

PET-CT aids in localizing the primary, staging, restaging, monitoring response to therapy and radiotherapy planning.

Neurology

Clinical indications for PET-CT are diagnosis and grading of tumors, tumor recurrence versus radiation

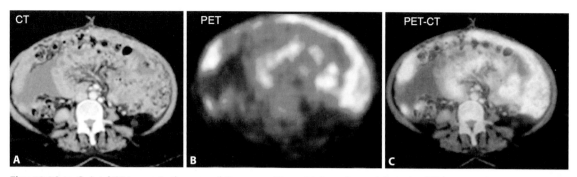

Figs 18.3A to C Axial CT image in the case of Ca ovary with multiple peritoneal deposits. Mild ascites also noted; (A) Post FDG injection PET; (B) PET-CT; and (C) image shows increased tracer uptake suggestive of peritoneal metastases (*For color version, see Plate 4*)

necrosis, seizure focus identification, dementias, brain injury, depression, schizophrenia, movement disorders with 18F-dopa, infection, and substance abuse. Thymidine and methionine are other tracers used in neurology.

Cardiology

Metabolic scan is gold standard in assessing cardiac viability (Thallium SPECT is more widely used for viability imaging). Perfusion scan is useful in detection of CAD-analogous to MP-SPECT with reported higher sensitivity and specificity with O-15, NH3 or Rubidium tracers. It aids information regarding coronary arteries, stenotic lesions and knowing about the hemodynamic significance of the same identified on CTCA.

Tuberculosis, Inflammatory Condition and Immunodeficiency Diseases

Infectious and noninfectious inflammatory conditions may demonstrate high FDG uptake. Elevated FDG accumulation in inflammatory tissues is related to increased glucose metabolism by the stimulated inflammatory cells, macrophage proliferation, and healing. In the patients with suspected infection and no known history of cancer, FDG PET may be quite useful for imaging localization of infectious disease. In difficult clinical cases the differentiation of FDG uptake in cancer versus an infectious or inflammatory lesion may become possible using sophisticated methods such as kinetic analysis and dual or more time-point PET scans. FDG PET has also been used in the imaging evaluation of patients with pyrexia of unknown origin (PUO).

One major area of recent interest has been in the evaluation of patients with suspected osteomyelitis and infected limb prosthesis implants.

There is increasing role of PET-CT in tuberculosis and immunodeficiency patients. It is important in immunodeficient patients to rule out lymphoma which is growing significantly, for this PET-CT guided biopsy could be the ultimate choice to differentiate between opportunistic infections versus lymphomas. Subsequent follow-up of the case should be done to assess the response to the therapy

FDG PET avoids many of the disadvantages of current techniques used in the imaging evaluation of patients with infectious and inflammatory diseases and provides a high degree of diagnostic accuracy in these clinical settings.

19

Magnetic Resonance-Positron Emission Tomography

Chandan Mishra

Magnetic resonance imaging (MRI) and positron emission tomography (PET) offer complementary functionality and sensitivity. Simultaneous acquisition provides a hybrid technology that is superior to the sum of its parts. MRI gives structural details and provides high soft tissue resolution images whereas PET uses a radioactive tracer in the body to obtain functional information of a particular organ or system, locate metastasis, recurrence of tumors and help in determining the effectiveness of treatment in malignant diseases. However PET gives molecular detail but fails to give anatomical information. The combined capability of MR-PET has been developed while PET evaluates the metabolic aspects and MRI gives high resolution anatomical information.

Different designs are available for combined MR-PET systems. Separate operations in different rooms are suggested as a low-budget approach to combined MR/PET; however, several practical challenges exist. An alternative approach to combine MR and PET information is to use a PET and an MR in tandem with a joined table platform. A second approach exploits the potential of solid-state light detectors (APDs) to allow the development of an MR-compatible PET detector insert that can be used inside a standard MR scanner.

A third, and most challenging approach, is with a PET insert that fit into a whole-body MR offering simultaneous MR/PET acquisitions (Figs 19.1A and B). It has unique workflow and acquisition benefits:

- *Better time management:* The simultaneous acquisition of PET and MR image reduces overall time for a PET/MR examination.
- *Better PET data:* With the time required to conduct an MR examination being optimized for PET data acquisition, the resultant quality of image is high.
- *Better infrastructural solution:* Installation requires a single standard dimension MR room, a single cooling system and single operating console room, reducing the infrastructural requirements.

- *Better patient comfort:* Reduces the MR and PET scan to a single pass through the machine.
- *Better patient management:* With a shorter overall imaging time, a higher patient throughput with optimal patient scheduling can be achieved.

Benefits of MRI-PET over CT-PET include

- The MRI provides superior soft-tissue contrast
- Cross evaluation of multiple imaging biomarkers. MR Spectroscopy, Diffusion imaging, Perfusion imaging, and functional MRI (fMRI) provide concurrent functional information with PET providing metabolic information. This improves your ability to accurately detect and stage disease, plan and optimize therapy selection and finally monitor treatment and follow-up.
- No radiation exposure from the MR will significantly reduce overall dose and prevent long term cell damage to patients undergoing repeated studies for therapy monitoring and/or follow-up.
- PET-MRI can differentiate tumor recurrence from fibrosis following radiotherapy.

NEURO APPLICATIONS OF MAGNETIC RESONANCE IMAGING-POSITRON EMISSION TOMOGRAPHY

It is used in detection and staging of gliomas and identification of areas with critical neurofunction around tumors, important for neurosurgery planning. In these cases MR Spectroscopy can be correlated with regional metabolic PET data (Fig. 19.2).

Simultaneous data acquisition of PET and MR allows the addition of kinetic, functional and metabolic information for real-time multimodality imaging, e.g. in solid tumors using diffusion weighted MRI and kinetic constants from PET.

Hybrid MR-PET provides insights into critical treatment approaches in neurosciences such as effect of deep brain stimulation showing metabolism in

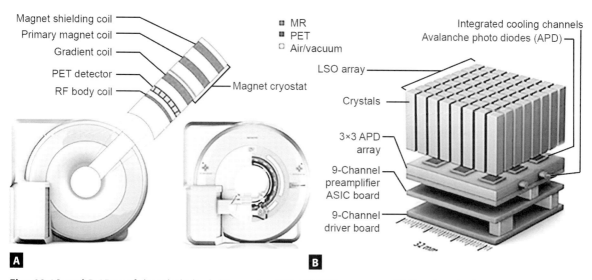

Figs 19.1A and B View of the whole-body Biograph mMR, MR-PET prototype: (A) Showing the basic components of the system where the PET detector ring is placed between the RF coil and the RF body coil; (B) Configuration of the detector block consisting of 8×8 LSO crystals read-out by a matrix of 3×3 APDs. LSO is Lutetium Oxyorthosilicate and ASIC is detector stack (*For color version, see Plate 4*)

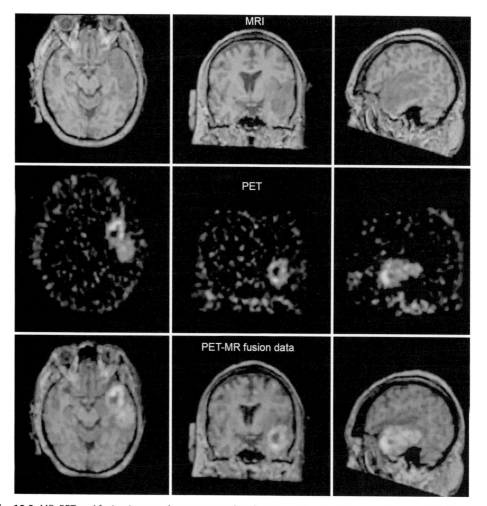

Fig. 19.2 MR, PET and fusion images demonstrates the glioma proliferation (*Courtesy:* Siemens AG, Germany) (*For color version, see Plate 5*)

defined regions together with the connecting neuronal tracts (from Diffusion Tensor MRI).

ONCOLOGICAL APPLICATIONS OF MAGNETIC RESONANCE IMAGING-POSITRON EMISSION TOMOGRAPHY

Melanoma management: MRI is significant for active disease whereas FDG-PET provides information about therapy response.

Nonsmall cell lung cancer: Evaluation with MRI is useful for brain and hepatic lesions whereas lymph node status and soft tissue metastases is detected by PET scans.

Liver metastasis: From primaries at GI tract, lung, pancreas etc. will benefit from the superior detection and characterization of MRI where in PET have limitations due to normal liver tissue uptake (Fig. 19.3).

Neuroendocrine tumors: Metastasis to liver sometimes are not visualized using labeled radio-nucleotides but contrast enhanced MRI can add significant information.

Pelvic masses: Prostate and cervical cancer for evaluating bone status in case of metastasis (Figs 19.4A to C).

Combination of MRI and PET providing fast imaging protocols without additional radiation exposure appears to be a very attractive imaging solution for evaluation of several cardiovascular

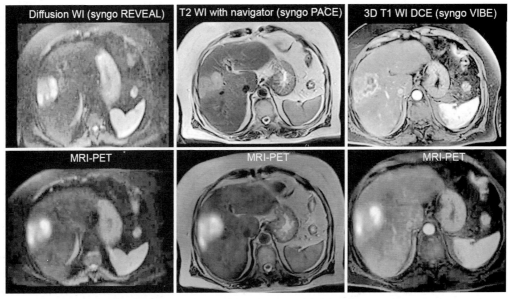

Fig. 19.3 Simultaneous acquisition PET with multiple MRI information showing better characterization of hepatic lesion (*For color version, see Plate 6*)

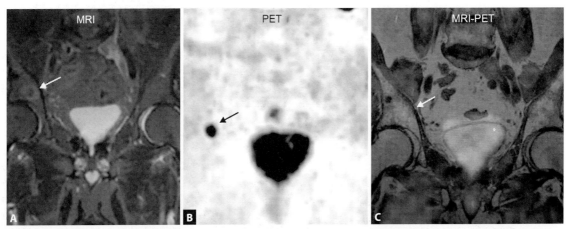

Figs 19.4A to C Simultaneous MR and PET support detection and monitoring of prostate cancer where whole-body MR offers high contrast to identify small and diffuse metastasis and PET enables superb lesion detection and differentiation (A) whole body MR; (B) Choline PET; (C) simultaneous MR and PET (*For color version, see Plate 6*)

diseases. Assessment of infarction and viability with more detailed risk assessment by combining glucose uptake (jeopardized myocardium) and delayed enhancement (irreversible scar). Left ventricle function with perfusion, metabolic or molecular imaging will improve stratification of heart failure. Also possibility to combine anatomy (plaque burden, luminal obstruction) with hemodynamic consequences (ischemia) for CAD will increase the therapeutic confidence.

Whole-body MR-PET creates a synergy to reach beyond the capabilities with unlocking new applications, defying the progress of disease, reinvent the future of disease management. MR-PET simultaneous imaging will open avenues like combining dynamic PET acquisition with functional MRI. Combination of various MR spectroscopy procedures with PET helps in broadening insight into the complex metabolic changes caused by brain diseases.

20

Single-photon Emission Computed Tomography

Sikandar Shaikh

Functional imaging methods include single-photon emission computed tomography (SPECT), positron emission tomography (PET), and magnetic resonance spectroscopy (MRS). These methods assess regional differences in the biochemical status of tissues.

In SPECT, functional measurements are performed by administering the patient with a radiopharmaceutical that is accumulation response to its biochemical characteristics. By design, the radiopharmaceutical has a targeted action, allowing it to be imaged to evaluate specific physiological processes in the body. Because the amount of radioactivity that can be administered internally to the patient is limited by considerations of radiation dose, radionuclide images inherently have poor photon statistics, are produced with only modest spatial resolution, and require relatively long scan times.

This technique, often called dual modality imaging, physically combines a SPECT system with a CT scanner, using a common patient table, computer and gantry so that both the X-ray and radionuclide image data are acquired sequentially without removing the patient from the scanner. This technique thereby produces anatomical and functional images with the patient in the same position and during a single procedure, which simplifies the image registration and fusion processes. X-ray images provide detailed anatomical information that helps the physician to differentiate normal radionuclide uptake from that indicating disease and to help localize disease sites within the body.

GAMMA CAMERA

A gamma camera is a system of one or more detectors, linked to an acquisition computer. In front of each detector is a collimator, which projects an image of the radioactive distribution onto the crystal. These images are analogous to planar X-rays. The crystal converts the incoming gamma-ray signal to a light signal, which is detected by an array of photomultiplier tubes (PMTs).

The PMT signals are processed to form the image which is stored on an acquisition computer. Images are downloaded to a processing computer.

X-ray scatter from the patient that has the potential to reach and possibly damage the radionuclide detectors, which are designed for the relatively low photon rate encountered in radionuclide imaging. To avoid this possibility, the radionuclide detector in a dual-modality system is typically offset in the axial direction from the plane of the X-ray source and detector. This distance can be relatively small when a low-dose 140 kV, 1-mA X-ray tube is used, but can be 60 cm or more when a diagnostic CT scanner is coupled to a modern PET scanner operated without septa.

In first-generation SPECT systems, the SPECT detectors and CT imaging chain were mounted on the same rotating platform and were used sequentially while rotated around the patient. This limited the rotational speed of the X-ray and radionuclide imaging chains to approximately 20 seconds per rotation, but also had the advantage that it could be performed using a gantry similar to that used with a conventional scintillation camera. Second-generation SPECT systems include high-performance diagnostic CT subsystems. This requires the heavy SPECT detectors to be mounted on a separate rotating platform from the CT imaging chain, which is rotated at speeds of 0.25 to 0.4 seconds per revolution. While this design obviously increases the performance of the CT subsystem, it also increases the cost and complexity of the gantry.

In currently available dual-modality scanners, the computer systems are well integrated in terms of system control, data acquisition, image reconstruction, image display and data processing and analysis. The CT data have to be calibrated so that the data can be used as an attenuation map to correct the radionuclide data for photon attenuation. For physician review, the CT and radionuclide data are registered and presented with the radionuclide image as a color overlay on the gray-scale CT image. Available software functions allow the operator to utilize the dual-modality data in correcting, viewing and interpreting, and are therefore important design elements in modern dual-modality imaging systems.

Technetium-99m (99mTc)-Sestamibi SPECT for Parathyroid Imaging

The parathyroid scan uses sestamibi (or MIBI for short) for localization of parathyroid adenomas (PTA) in the neck. It is facilitated by visualization of the thyroid gland in the early phase of the study and is improved with occasional SPECT-MIBI. SPECT, however, contributes to precise PTA localization and to planning of the surgical strategy in patients with deep-seated adenomas in the neck, or in those with distorted cervical anatomy following neck surgery or with concomitant multinodular goitre (MNG) or ectopic adenomas. The major role of SPECT is in patients with an ectopic PTA and in patients after prior failed surgery. The 3-D presentation of an adenoma on SPECT in the presence of known anatomical structures provides an optimized surgical road map towards easy accessibility of the PTA, a shorter invasive procedure, and a higher success rate.

SPECT need not necessarily be applied to patients with a well-defined cervical PTA on planar MIBI scintigraphy prior to initial surgery, in the absence of associated medical conditions of the neck. Combined functional and morphologic information provided by SPECT appears to be a promising prerequisite tool for minimally invasive surgery in patients with primary hyperparathyroidism with a more complicated clinical background or in a difficult anatomic location.

131-Iodine SPECT for Thyroid Cancer Imaging

Use of 131-Iodine SPECT fusion imaging, especially after the administration of a relatively high treatment dose, will provide clinically relevant diagnostic information in a high proportion of patients with recurrent or metastatic thyroid cancer. It is most useful in clarifying the location of foci of increased uptake seen on planar images and differentiating physiologic radioiodine activity from uptake in malignant sites, thus permitting the avoidance of additional, at times invasive, diagnostic procedures. The improved diagnostic interpretation provided by the availability of combined SPECT images has been reported to change management decisions in at least one-third of patients with thyroid cancer (Figs 20.1A to F).

123-Iodine MIBG SPECT for Tumor Imaging

Single-photon emission computed tomography moves nuclear medicine procedures closer to one of the ultimate goals of functional imaging: namely, the quantitative measurement of radionuclide concentration. This appears to be of particular significance for MIBG (meta-iodo-benzyl-guanidine), when labeled with 131-I, is being used for treatment of advanced stage neuroendocrine tumors and neuroblastoma. The ability to precisely determine the percent of injected dose of MIBG taken up by the tumor and the effective half-life of the drug, using tracer doses of either the 123-I or 131-I labeled agent, may allow for better treatment-tailoring in the individual patient, and may potentially lead to higher chances for response to this therapeutic modality.

111-Indium Octreotide SPECT for Neuroendocrine Tumor Imaging

111-Inoctreotide is used for the detection of neuro-endocrine tumors. The clinical utility of 111-In-octreotide as an imaging agent to identify somatostatin receptor expression in tumors, both neuroendocrine and nonneuroendocrine, as well as in granulomas and autoimmune processes based on the accumulation of activated inflammatory cells that contained somatostatin receptors.

This agent is used for *in vivo* scintigraphic detection of pituitary tumors, carcinoid, gastrinoma, islet cell tumors, medullary thyroid carcinoma, pheochromocytoma, and paraganglioma, as well as neuroblastoma, small cell lung carcinoma, Hodgkin's and non-Hodgkin's lymphoma, active sarcoid and tuberculous lesions, hyperfunctioning thyroid glands, and clinically active Graves' ophthalmopathy.

Bone SPECT in Oncology

Technetium-99m (99mTc) methylene diphosphonate (MDP) is currently the most widely used radio-pharmaceutical in bone scintigraphy. The phosphonate compounds bind to bone by chemisorption to the hydroxyapatite crystal. 99mTc decays to 99Tc by releasing a 140 keV gamma ray, which is efficiently detected by a gamma camera. Bone scintigraphy reflects skeletal metabolic activity. Skeletal diphosphonate uptake is influenced by blood flow and osteoblastic activity related to new bone formation.

Bone scintigraphy therefore has a high sensitivity for the detection of bone metastases, mainly osteoblastic lesions and becomes positive before plain radiographs, due to the appearance of focal areas of increased bone turnover in response to tumor growth (Figs 20.2A to C).

Changes in bone formation of as little as 5% to 15% can be detected. Lesions showing only bone resorption may be detected as photopenic regions.

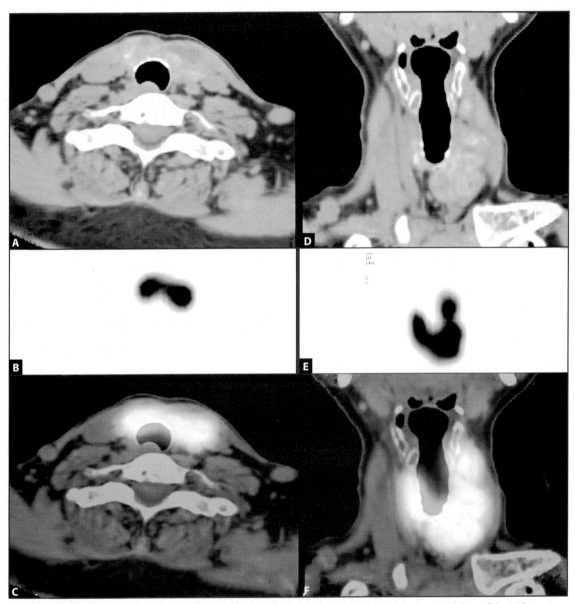

Figs 20.1A to F Axial and coronal CT images of neck (A and D) showing multiple nodules in both lobes of thyroid, more on the left. On administration of 131I, it shows increased uptake in thyroid gland seen on fusion images of SPECT (B, C, E and F) (*For color version, see Plate 7*)

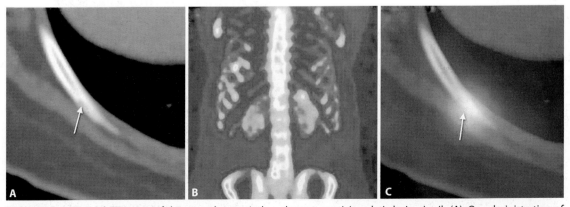

Figs 20.2A to C Axial CT image of thorax on bone window shows a suspicious lytic lesion in rib (A). On administration of Technetium-99m methylene diphosphonate (MDP) it showed increased uptake in rib, seen on fusion images suggestive of metastatic lesion (B and C) (*For color version, see Plate 8*)

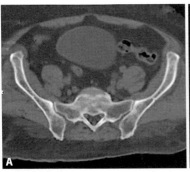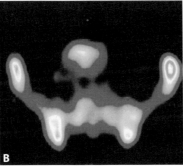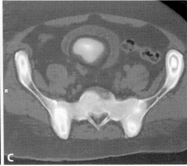

Figs 20.3A to C Axial CT section at level of iliac bones does not show any obvious abnormality in a case of prostate cancer (A). On administration of 111In capromab pendetide it showed increased uptake in prostate gland and left anterior superior iliac spine, seen on fusion images, s/o metastatic lesion (B and C) (*For color version, see Plate 8*)

Computed tomography is a highly sensitive method for evaluating cortical and trabecular bone, being able to assess minimal bone changes in an early stage of destruction and also to classify lesions at risk for fracture or diagnose spine misalignment, because of the capacity of multiplanar reformats.

SPECT Imaging for Prostate Cancer

111In capromab pendetide is a radiolabeled murine monoclonal antibody. 111In capromab pendetide scintigraphy has been shown to be superior to CT and MRI in identifying metastatic prostate carcinoma. The technique is complimentary to the Gleason score, PSA, and clinical staging in the assessment of prognosis.

SPECT appears to be the optimal modality to detect occult metastases in high-risk patients with presumed localized disease. Results of 111In capromab pendetide SPECT imaging may influence the choice and planning of the appropriate therapy approach (Figs 20.3A to C).

67Gallium SPECT in Imaging of Lymphoma

SPECT can be useful in the precise identification and characterization of disease sites at various locations. In the region of the head and neck, gallium SPECT can be of value in the diagnosis of lymphoma of the thyroid, a rare extranodal site of disease and in its differentiation from involvement of adjacent cervical adenopathy. In the chest, SPECT can define the precise relationship of gallium uptake to one of the various adjacent thoracic structures. Precise differentiation of hilar from mediastinal involvement may alter disease stage. SPECT can differentiate between paramediastinal lung lesion (indicative of stage IV disease) and mediastinal adenopathy, as well as between peripheral lung involvement and a rib lesion.

SPECT in the Evaluation of Infection

67Gallium citrate (Ga) is currently used for the investigation of fever of unknown origin, acute or chronic osteomyelitis and the diagnosis of infections in immuno-compromised patients. In assessment of musculoskeletal infection, Ga scintigraphy is usually performed in conjunction with 99mTc methylene diphosphonate (MDP) bone scintigraphy.

RADIOLABELED LEUKOCYTES

Labelled WBC imaging using either 99mTc- or 111In has been shown to perform excellently in detecting acute and chronic infections. This test has become the nuclear medicine modality of choice in a variety of clinical settings when the suspicion of an infectious process exists. Clinical indications for labelled leukocytes scintigraphy include osteomyelitis, especially in cases where infected joint prosthesis or post-traumatic osteomyelitis is suspected. WBC scintigraphy has also been advocated for assessment of suspected vascular graft infections, diabetic foot, and abdominal infections.

ADDITIONAL RADIOLABELED MOLECULES FOR INFECTION IMAGING

There have been many innovations in nuclear medicine imaging of infections since the first use of Ga, a tracer with a nonspecific mechanism of uptake in infection sites.

Over the years, more specific agents (such as labeled WBC) and even receptor specific proteins (such as antigranulocyte and antibody fragments) have been introduced.

The cumulative knowledge and better understanding of the biochemical processes of infection have led to the development of labeled receptor-specific small proteins and peptides.

21

Picture Archiving and Communication System

Parvez Seikh

Picture archiving and communication system (PACS) stores and transmits images electronically over the internet or local area network (LAN) and viewed using suitable computer consoles and devices. The images can be accessed either within the hospital premises or at remote locations outside the hospital. PACS eliminates the need for maintaining hard copies of radiology films and reports by creating a filmless environment for easy and timely access to retrieve images and reports.

Radiology department has been a pioneer in developing PACS to its current high standards. In early 1980's the concept of using electronic storage and transmission of radiology images and reports was introduced. Due to prohibitive costs and technology issues PACS could not find many takers to start with. As the core technology of PACS rapidly progressed due to advances in technology, the capabilities of PACS improved potentially. For instance, the hard disk storage options improved, more images can be stored, retrieved and transmitted faster.

Presently PACS worldwide has become an indispensable workflow system in modern hospitals. Ideally CAT6 networking cables should be installed to maintain adequate transfer of data and images. Some hospitals continue to use outdated CAT5 networking cables; in such instances the PACS data transmission is slow. In addition to the networking cables appropriate routers, switches and firewalls are equally important for a secure and efficient network.

PICTURE ARCHIVING AND COMMUNICATION SYSTEM

- Imaging equipment like X-ray and fluoroscopy, diagnostic ultrasound, CT scan, MRI, mammography PET scan and SPECT images.
- Secured network for transmission of patient information, preferably broadband internet.

- Workstations that have compatible hardware and software to retrieve the images and data for interpretation and reporting.
- Data storage archives on computer server to store images and reports.
- Server for backup copies at a remote location so that these images can be retrieved when the main PACS server is under maintenance care.

The PACS workflow system includes image acquisition; digital images are modified to PACS compatible images, data transfer to a central computer server, with appropriate data storage and archiving, remote access for viewing the images, providing support to clinicians. Some hospital might still use analogue radiographs that need to be scanned and converted into digital images for PACS. Its maintenance team should be readily available 24/7 to tackle software and hardware breakdown.

SOME TECHNICAL FEATURES OF PICTURE ARCHIVING AND COMMUNICATION SYSTEM

- The hospital information system (HIS) server contains patient data and request for investigations (Flow chart 21.1), it is vendor specific and should be compatible with PACS.
- The Radiology Information System (RIS) contains the modality requested (Fig. 21.1), this server is integrated with PACS.
- All the peripherals like external digital video decoders (DVD) writers, external universal serial bus (USB) ports, data backup and printing devices are integrated with PACS.
- Fine tuning of PACS with hospital digital imaging and communications in medicine (DICOM) is done for compressing images and reports, adjusting optimum speed of transmission, proxy IP (internet protocol) for networks, server functioning, remote data server for backups for image retrieval.

Flow chart 21.1 Workflow between HIS and PACS

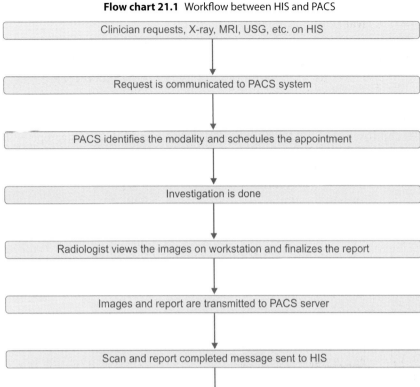

Note: Hospital information system (HIS) might use vendor specific software and operating system platform different from picture archiving and communication system (PACS)

Radiology information system workflow

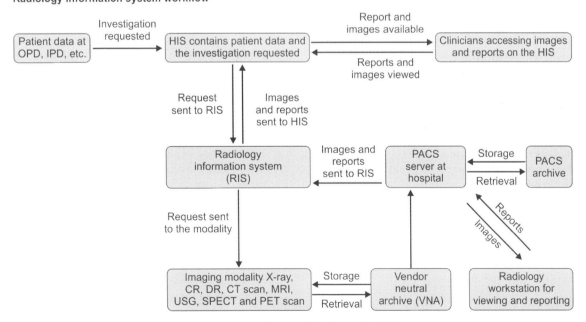

Fig. 21.1 Vendor neutral archive with PACS

- PACS is a web based system so it can be accessed wherever internet is available, it is hardware independent.
- Viewer can be installed on any operating systems like Linux, Mac or Windows for the radiologist to interpret them. PACS can support a wide range of mobile devices through Web Access to DICOM Objects (WADO) server. Mobile devices like iPhone, iPad, Android system based phones and tablets are compatible with PACS.
- Voice recognition system is integrated in PACS which eliminates the manual transmission of reports with improve efficiency.
- The reporting formats and templates according to the HIS are uploaded on PACS. Digital signatures are available for reporting purposes. After a report has been saved and finalized the reporting software locks the report and no changes can be made. The report is then available for the clinicians.
- HL7 translator software integrates several PACS and radiology information systems. It is an interfaceware that coverts several formats from various sources to a standard format to view images and reports. It is more useful in Teleradiology to ensure compatibility between various PACS systems and helps to avoid errors. HL7 translator can improve the efficiency and serve as productivity enhancing tool.

Vendor Neutral Archive

PACS stores images in a vendor specific format of compression and storage, this can be a minor problem when the hospital decides to upgrade or switch to a newer PACS system. Vendor neutral archive (VNA) is a neutral format for storing the images directly from the imaging modality into the hospital computer server. Images are then transmitted from the VNA to PACS system. In this way images can be stored in the hospital database and viewed/retrieved when necessary (Fig. 21.2).

Current approach

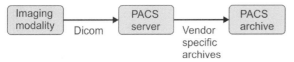

Newer approach of using vendor neutral archive (VNA) with PACS

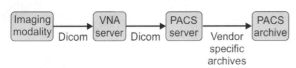

Fig. 21.2 Radiology information workflow

Advantages of PACS

- Fast and easy access to images and reports in the hospital which improves patient care. Radiology images can be transmitted from peripheral clinics to hospitals for reporting the MRI, PET and CT scans due to lack of availability of radiologist at the clinic.
- No accumulation of paper reports and image films, PACS can store them electronically, saves time and space. This can prove cost-effective in the long term planning.
- Images can be sent for second opinion/consultation using internet within the country and abroad.
- PACS can be connected to Teleradiology software, radiologists can access the hospital PACS using their personal computers, iPads and mobile phones.

Drawbacks of PACS

- PACS is an expensive investment initially but the costs can be recovered over a 5-year-period.
- Important to train doctors, technicians, receptionists, other hospital staff to use PACS effectively.
- PACS eliminates the need for hard copy of radiology films and reports, the result is a filmless Radiology department, this might take sometime for the department to get used to this situation.
- Data might get lost due to some software or hardware problem. Storage of data at some remote location is very essential to retrieve the data.
- PACS have many different features and configurations to suit the unique needs of each hospital. Vendors try and promote their PACS products to hospitals. Some extra features quoted the vendors might not be required by the hospital. Ideally trial version of PACS should be installed for atleast a month in Radiology department before any major decision is taken to purchase it.
- Radiology data images and reports might consume significant bandwidth of existing Local area network (LAN) or internet traffic within the hospital. The PACS system selected should not overburden the existing networks in the hospital.
- Dedicated maintenance is needed to keep PACS operational. It involves addressing and overcoming issues related to widely varied networks, creating secure virtual private network tunnels (VPN), configuring multiple firewalls on network and testing digital imaging and communications in medicine (DICOM) transfers.

Training of Hospital Staff

On-site PACS training for hospital staff is essential to improve productivity and efficiency of PACS. Hospital staff should be given hands on training to make them comfortable using PACS systems. PACS can adapt to the unique requirements of different Radiology departments. Ideally after the complete installation of PACS, the radiology department staff should be confident to compress images data and reports, transfer data efficiently so that productivity of PACS starts from the first day of installation. PACS vendors can also provide web-based updates and meetings to address issues regarding the usage of PACS similar to distance learning modules; interactive web sessions with periodic reviews are helpful.

Troubleshooting, Maintenance and Warranty Issues

Periodic troubleshooting, updating the software, installing new peripherals, server upgrades, retrieving lost files and regular maintenance checks ensure PACS functioning smoothly. Some examples include defragmentation of workstation memory, clearing the cache on workstations, updating antivirus software, clearing the computer registry. A dedicated and qualified PACS administrator with IT support team should be readily available at a short notice to resolve any glitches. The vendor should ideally provide warranty for the initial three years after installation of PACS. Annual renewal should be available at lower cost from fourth year onwards after installation. Any additional hardware upgrades or replacements for PACS server needs to be considered should also be taken into consideration as some radiology equipment might not be covered in warranty.

Changing or Switching to New PACS Vendor

The hospital might want to change to a new PACS vendor due to various reasons like obsolete software and hardware, requirement of the radiology department have changed, maintenance problems, etc. The transition to install a new PACS must be smooth and effective, also it is essential to training the staff all over again. There must be some specific features or functions in the new PACS which the existing PACS in the hospital cannot offer. It might be beneficial to discuss the problems faced in the new PACS with their existing customer base.

Quality Assurance in PACS

It is an essential aspect of PACS, from a clinical perspective. Image quality is important for any hospital using PACS. Basic system design and PACS training for staff can help to improve image quality. The quality of images viewed on PACS should be the same on different consoles used in hospital. The PACS images should in no way be inferior to hard copies of radiology images. PACS system has features to adjust the images for better viewing like contrast, brightness, flipping the image, zooming the image, add annotations and remarks to the images. Default settings can be applied to images so that each incoming images in PACS system are automatically optimized for viewing purposes. All PACS display devices such as computer consoles should undergo periodic Quality assurance tests for monitoring PACS performance. If for some reason a PACS workstation does not meet all the requirements of the PACS, that machine should be labeled as non-suitable for PACS and explanation submitted to the hospital. PACS images that are not adequate for viewing should be kept in a separate folder in PACS so that they can be evaluated later by PACS maintenance team.

Computer Console Specifications

The LCD of computer console should operate at optimal resolution (Table 21.1), this is to ensure that the ratio between screen pixels and screen resolution is 1:1 at all times.

Images where the image resolution is more than three megapixels are helpful in image interpretation.

PACS (Fig. 21.3) is a combination of hardware and software dedicated to short-and long-term storage, retrieval, management, distribution and presentation of images. The purpose of PACS is to improve efficiency by creating a filmless environment while maintaining or improving diagnostic ability of radiology department. PACS acts like an electronic gateway system using a dedicated PACS computer server. PACS uses both local area network (LAN) and internet, data management system that controls the workflow on a network and storage devices for image archives. The input of PACS can be from digital or analog sources, the input from analog sources are first converted into digital format before they can be sent to PACS system. Display devices for PACS-like computer consoles, voice dictation devices, keyboard and mouse are needed to view the images and data. The cost effectiveness of PACS must be proven before installing it

Table 21.1 PACS workstation console requirements suggested by Royal College of Radiologists (UK)

	Minimum	Recommended
Screen resolution (native pixel array)	>1280 × 1024 (appx. 1.3 megapixels)	> 1500 × 2000 (appx. 3 megapixels)
Screen size (viewable diagonal)	17 inch	20 inch
Maximum luminance	170 cd/m^2	> 500 cd/m^2
Luminance ratio	> 250:1	> 500 :1
Grayscale calibration	Within 10% of grayscale	Calibrated to grayscale
Video display interface	Digital analog	Digital video interface (DVI)

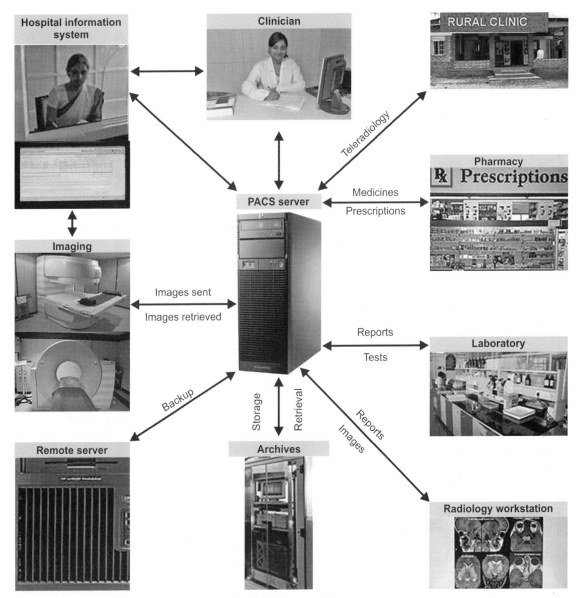

Fig. 21.3 PACS workflow

in hospitals, initial setup is usually expensive. Training of radiology staff is important to effectively utilize PACS. Maintenance is done by a dedicated team of IT professionals. Switching or upgrading to a new vendor must be carefully done after weighting the pros and cons. VNA can store images directly from the imaging modality and transmit the images to the PACS system. Quality assurance testing and monitoring is important to maintain image resolution for interpreting radiology images.

22

Planning of Radiology Department

Raunaklaxmi Laul

Since the discovery of X-rays by Roentgen in 1895 radiology has come a long way. No other medical science has seen such explosive development. This facilitates the need for appropriate planning and management of radiology departments as it takes into accounts a hoard of modalities which require careful installation, sophisticated handling, and effective management. In addition to this there is also need for appropriate protective measures to be taken to protect the staff, patients and the general public from the radiation hazards arising due to the use of radiations. Thus a careful, well-considered planning is needed for the effective working of a radiology department with effective accommodation of any future developments. The planning strategy has been described under following headings:

- Modalities
- Planning considerations and organization of department
- Safety considerations and protective measures.
- Housing modalities for imaging equipment
- Maintenance and management.

MODALITIES

The radiology department works on basis of variety of modalities incorporated in one department with the objective of

- Providing high quality imaging service
- Establishment and confirmation of clinical diagnosis
- Providing high quality therapeutic radiology services
- And research and training.

Thus, the various imaging modalities used are:

- X-ray machines
- Fluoroscopy machine for special procedures
- Ultrasound machine with Doppler
- Computed tomography (CT Scan)
- Magnetic resonance imaging (MR)
- Mammography
- Digital subtraction angiography (DSA).

The planning of the radiology department is based upon the daily patients flow, not on the total capacity of the hospital. That means, if up to 100 X-rays needs to be done daily one X-ray machine is sufficient, but in the setting requiring more than 100 X-rays daily at least two X-ray machines are required. Similarly, one ultrasound machine is enough if daily up to 80 sonographies needs to be done, for more sonographies one more machine will be required. So, the strategy for planning the radiology department is influenced by the workload.

PLANNING CONSIDERATIONS

Planning of the department should include three critical steps:

1. Physical planning
2. Strategic planning
3. Visionary planning.

Physical Planning

The physical planning of the department takes into consideration the area, location and other basic points:

- *Location:* The radiology department should be preferably located on the ground floor which facilitates easy access to the patients and also should be well connected to the OPD, emergency and the indoor services. The department should be located away from maternity and pediatric wards to prevent radiation hazards.
- *Size*: The size usually depends on the hospital size and the number of machines to be installed but it should also be adequate to permit appropriate ventilation and accommodate radiation protective barriers.
- *Area:* It should include administrative, ancillary and auxiliary area in addition to the Functional area which houses the machinery.
- *Administrative area:* Includes reception with patient registration counter and announcing system, Patient waiting, offices of head of the

department and other radiologists on staff, offices for nursing and technical staff.

- *Ancillary area:* It includes film library with record room, store for supplies, and ample circulation space for patients, staff and trolleys. It should also accommodate toilets and changing rooms for staff and patients and seminar room for case discussions.
- *Auxiliary area:* Includes patient preparation room and reporting desks.
- *Functional area:* It actually houses the necessary machines and hence should be well shielded and all the possible protective measures are needed to be taken to ensure protection of workers and patients in accordance with the guidelines of atomic energy regulatory board. It should include the X-ray rooms with adjacent fluoroscopy room for special procedures. A mammography unit and the DSA unit should also be adjacent to X-ray rooms so that all radiation causing modalities are segregated together. CT and MR are to be installed in such a way that they can have a common working and reporting console for the ease of the patient and the radiologist. Ultrasound and Doppler should be incorporated together and should have separate toilet facility for patients. In addition to this a central printing and processing room should be created with adequate implantation of PACS to facilitate X-ray and procedure film processing and printing and should be connected by local area network to CT and MR console for film printing. There should also be rooms for report typing separately for the X-ray, CT and MR, Ultrasound and nuclear imaging modalities.

All these rooms should be well shielded between actual machinery and the staff area to prevent radiation hazards with and optimal distance of at least 3 meters between the machine and the control panel. All the machine housing areas and control panels should have a three phase (40 kilo watts) electrical supply with double earthing and back-up for the central processing units with generators. It should ideally be separate from the main supply of the rest of the hospital. The switch should be located at a height of 1270 mm from the finished floor with a copper strip below the main switch. Voltage should be ideally of 415 volts, with 50 Hz frequency and 0.36 ohms of resistance from phase to phase. The generator should be 2 pulse generator to run the sophisticated machinery in case of an emergency in power failure. Wiring used should be of size 12 square millimeters made up of copper. There should be air conditioning of the department centrally for the administrative, auxiliary and ancillary area with separate air conditioning with temperature control for CT and MR, nuclear imaging area, X-ray, mammography, procedure room and USG room. There should be adequate air-conditioning for the digital processing and printing room. If the department needs to have provisions for teleradiology then a separate console has to be made with internet access. In addition to this adequate imaging soft wares with local network connection are to be connected in all the radiologists' rooms to provide easy reporting, it should have connection to all consoles for aggregation of all types of images on the computers. The book and film library should also preferably digitalized and include the seminar room. The store should be well equipped with all the required accessories like digital cassettes, X-ray, CT and MR films, lead aprons, gloves and shields, printing papers, envelopes for film and report dispatch, stationary, printer cartridges, and cleaning material. The record room should be updated preferably weekly with all modality records arranged and kept separately. There should be some system in record arrangement so that a certain patient's record on a certain date can be found if required without problems. The department should be well lit and ventilated and kept clean to ensure healthy working environment.

The department should be adequately staffed, so that it should work smoothly. Staffing depends upon the work load, types and timings of the services provided. There should be a standard operating procedure for all categories of staff to ensure overall smooth organization and functioning. The staff should include:

- *Radiologists:* Head of department, senior and junior consultants, senior and junior residents.
- *Technical:* Supervisor, senior and junior technicians for all modalities, radiographers for processing and printing, assistants for ultrasound.
- *Nursing:* Sister in charge, both male and female staff nurses trained in patient preparation and emergency care.
- *Others:* Receptionist, typists, storekeeper, cleaning assistants and library attendant.
- The technicians should be well distributed to be available for working and emergency hours.

Strategic Planning

Strategic planning is an organization's process of defining its direction, and making decisions on allocating its resources to pursue this strategy. As radiology continues to grow, radiologists must preparing radiology for the future. Decisions in capital investments, diagnostic clinics, and payment and liability on loans will require the radiologists to develop and follow up managerial, interpersonal, and learning skills that were not as necessary in the past.

Visionary Planning

Visionary planning is thinking about the future or advancements in a creative and imaginative way. A person who is ahead of his time and who has a powerful plan for change in the future is an example of a visionary. This includes thinking critically and constructively about planning future work spaces. New approaches to radiology department design are illustrated by describing care environment and then examining the resultant facility requirements, the architecture is beyond the building design. Facilities programming is not only projecting departmental need for the near term but raising questions: why, why not, how, what, when, if's and but's be evaluated.

SAFETY CONSIDERATIONS AND PROTECTIVE MEASURES

Safety measures to be taken while installing a radiology department are based on the concept of ALARA which means as low as reasonably achievable radiation. Radiation protection has to be planned prior to the construction of the department and it should be according to the guidelines of radiation protection rule 1971 under atomic energy act 1962. The plan has to be submitted and approved by Atomic Energy Regulatory Board (AERB) at Bhabha Atomic Research Center, Mumbai. There should be awareness amongst the staff, patients and public regarding the radiation hazards and effective protective measures.

Radiation hazards can be:
- Deterministic effects which do not depend on radiation dosage
- Stochastic effects which depend on radiation dosage
- Somatic and genetic effects
- Acute and chronic effects.

Acute effects usually occur due to heavy dosage in short period of time, it consists of convulsions, headache, blurring of vision, nausea, vomiting, colicky abdominal pain, aplastic anemia, blood dyscrasias, and bone marrow depression.

Whereas chronic effects usually occur due to continuous short dose exposure. They can be loss of hair, burns, brittle nails, amputations, anemia, leukemia's, leukopenia, cataract, iridocyclitis, sterility, cancers, and mutations.

The overall planning of radiation protection should include:
- *Staff:* The distance between the control panel to regulate a machine and the actual machine should be at least 3 meters. Appropriate lead shielding has to done in all the areas housing radiation with lead equivalence of at least 1.5 cm. All staff members should be instructed to wear lead aprons, gloves, masks and gonadal and thyroidal shields. All personnel should also use the radiation monitoring devices like TLD badges.
- *Patients:* There should be adequate optimization of radiation dosage to patients by minimizing the area of exposure, use of appropriate devices to control scatter radiation and periodic quality control and calibration of machines. There should also be patient shielding with thyroid and gonad shielding and menstruating women should be subjected to radiation only after confirming that they are not pregnant.
- *Public:* There should be demarcation of the radioactive areas for public protection. Department should be located away from main traffic. The construction should be with brick and concrete walls at least 1.5 to 2 ft thick. Lead shielding of 1.5 mm equivalence should be done along all the external and internal walls. There should be signs indicating hazards and light signs to indicate ongoing of a procedure at all the necessary places. Radiation warning boards in light yellow color should be put on all the entrances to demarcate the departmental area. There should also adequate disposal of all radioactive and nuclear wastes.

HOUSING MODALITIES FOR IMAGING EQUIPMENT

Installation for radiation housing modalities (Fig. 22.1) like X-rays, fluoroscopy and IITV, mammography, CT should be in accordance with guidelines of AERB safety code made in 1986 which was revised to form the 'Medical diagnostic X-ray equipment and installations code' which has incorporated all the suggestions of International Commission of Radiation Protection (ICRP) guidelines. All the departments have to submit a layout of the rooms and then obtain a no objection certificate along with approval of Radiation Safety Officer before installation. The layout has to be send to AERB along with the prescribed form and the necessary fees to obtain approval. Also the list of personnel working, safety measures taken and TLD badges obtained has to be submitted. License for working is issued only after inspection of the site by the authority.

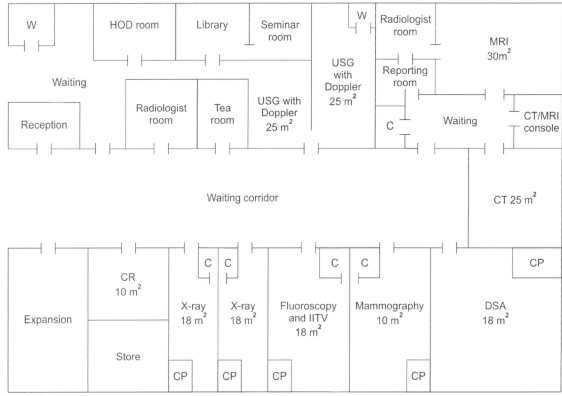

Fig. 22.1 Installation for radiation housing modalities

The license approved has to be renewed periodically. In case of obtaining radioactive isotopes for nuclear scanning additional approval has to obtained for periodic availability of radioactive material. There use has to be strictly monitored.

The required provisions for all the X-ray housing rooms are:

- Area should be such that it provides integrated facility of the unit, console and the waiting area. Also the room size should permit installation, use and servicing of equipment. As the radiation dose is inversely proportional to the area hence the rooms should be more than 18 square meters for diagnostic X-rays and more than 25 square meters for CT with no dimension less than 4 meters. There should be preferably one door located such that no primary beam falls on it.
- *Shielding:* It is required for all walls, ceiling and on the floor if the department is not on the ground floor. By keeping doors and windows away from the primary beam the cost for their shielding decreases leading to cost effectiveness. The walls on which the primary beam falls should be 35 cm thick and the walls on which it doesn't should be at least 23 cm thick. In addition to this lead shielding of

1.7 mm lead equivalence should be done on the walls and the doors and windows.

- Ventilation and natural light opening should at least be above a height of 2 feet from the finished floor.

Diagnostic X-ray, Fluoroscopy and IITV, Mammography, DSA Rooms

- *Diagnostic X-ray:* (500 milliamperes) a single room should be of 18 square meters size with no dimension less than 4 meters. The brick construction and shielding should be according to AERB guidelines mentioned above. Two adjacent rooms should have a brick partition with thickness of 23 cm. The tube housing should be constructed such that the leakage radiation through the protective tube in any direction is for not more than 100 square centimeters and it should not exceed 1 milligray per hour in a distance of 1 meter from the X-ray unit when the tube is operating at maximum kilovolt peak and tube current. There should be a visible mark on the tube housing to indicate plane of focus. Beam limiting collimators should be provided with beam filtration of at least 1.5 mm of aluminum. The cable length of the equipment should not be less than 3 m and the control panel should also be at least 2 m away with lead shielding of 1.7 mm lead equivalence. If the machine operates above 125 kVp then control panel should be constructed in a separate room. The control panel should indicate and enable control of exposure parameters and an identifiable indicator to show whether the X-ray beam is on/off. There should be an exposure switch to terminate the X-rays manually or after a preset timer. Radiation leakage from the transformer surface should not exceed 5 µGy in any direction in one hour. There should be adequate illumination control. The waiting area is demarcated and should have a conspicuous light to indicate ongoing of procedure. There should be a adjacent changing cubicle preferably in the room or adjacent to it with shielding of 1.5 mm lead equivalence.

- *Fluoroscopy and IITV:* The dimensions of the room should be same as the diagnostic X-ray room with similar tube housing. Beam filtration should not be less than 2 mm of aluminum. There should be a protective lead glass covering the fluorescent screen with a lead equivalence of 2 mm for units operating up to 100 kVp. For units operating at higher kVp lead thickness should be increased at a rate of 0.01 mm/kVp. Lead rubber flaps of 0.5 mm lead thickness should be suspended from bottom of the screen so that they overlap the fluoroscopy chair. X-ray tube and screen should be coupled and aligned to move together synchronously and the X-ray beam should pass through the center of screen in all positions. There should be field limiting diaphragms which are manually controlled so that when the diaphragm is fully opened and screen is at maximum distance there is still an unilluminated margin of at least 1 cm along all the edges of screen. Control knobs should have a shielding of 0.25 mm lead. Table top to focus distance should not be less than 30 cm and the table top exposure shall not exceed 5 µGy/min. There should be a control panel similar to that of X-ray unit. IITV (image intensifier television system) unit's tube housing is similar to that of general fluoroscopy. It should have a permanently incorporated protective barrier. The transmission through the barrier with the scatter should not exceed 20 µGy/hour at 10 cm distance from any accessible surface. Table top exposure should be less than 5 µGy/min and entrance exposure should not be greater than 3 µGy/exposure or 0.3 µGy/frame.

- *Mammography:* The required dimensions are 10 m² with 23 cm thick brick construction and 1.5 mm lead lined doors. The control panel in the room should have a 1.5 mm thick lead protective glass. The tube housing and shielding is similar to that of an X-ray unit. The beam limiting devices used should be such that at any target to receptor distance the beam size should not exceed beyond any edge of receptor. The transmitted dose should be less than 1 µGy/exposure at 5 cm beyond the breast support with no breast tissue present. Beam filtration should not be less than 0.03 mm of molybdenum. The cable length should be a minimum of 3 m with a control panel similar to that of X-ray room. The breast compression device should be such that it assures uniform thickness of the compressed breast with adjustable degree of compression.

- *DSA:* The minimum area requirement is of 18 m² with no single dimension less than 4 m and the control panel should have a lead viewing glass of thickness 2 mm. The construction should be of 23 cm thick brick wall with 2 mm lead lining the doors and windows. Most of the required structure is similar to that of an IITV room. The image intensifier used should have an intrinsic resolution of atleast 4 line pairs/mm at a modulation transfer value of 0.1. The video camera used should have a signal to noise ratio greater than 500:1. There should be proper use of personnel monitoring devices.

- *CT and MR:* CT and MR units should have a common console since most of the times a correlation and comparison is necessary between both the modalities. The total area comprising of both the units should be 150 m². As CT generates radiation, its layout has to be in accordance with the AERB guidelines. Area of 25 m² is used with 23 cm thick brick wall construction with 2 mm lead shielding on the walls for 100 kVp and additional 0.01 mm/kVp from 100 to 150 kVp and 2 mm thick lead shielding on the doors and windows. The console should have a 2 mm thick lead viewing glass. Tube housing is similar to that of X-ray rooms and the filter provided should be a bow-tie filter for both beam hardening and beam flattening. Visual indicators should be placed for control on console and on gantry to indicate scanning in progress. Space should be enough to facilitate the gantry tilt. Adequate warm up of the tube should be done and there should be warning signs put on the doors and the console to indicate warm-up in progress. There should be provision for oxygen support for patients and emergency drug tray.

The common console for CT and MR should have a 2 mm lead viewing glass on the side adjacent to CT and radiofrequency (RF) shielded wall and glass for the MR side. There should be a waiting area for patients especially those on oral dose of CT contrast with additional space for patient changing room, toilet and reception and doctor's room.

MR uses the technology of a high strength permanent magnet which generate magnetic field after passing electricity through magnetic coils which are bathed in cryogenic liquids like helium to make them superconducting. These magnets are to be shielded to allow MR scanners to be located in vicinity of objects sensitive to magnetic fields such as building structure, elevators, vehicles, etc. Shielding can be done by:

- *Radiofrequency (RF) shielding:* Done to prevent incidental RF energies from entering the scanning room and disrupting image acquisition process. Construction of thin sheets of copper foils is done on all the walls, ceiling and flooring and all the doors and windows. All the power cables exhaust and piping should pass through RF shielded enclosure and special RF filters.

- *Passive shielding:* Done in addition to RF shielding in forms of sheets of laminated steel alloy and is usually done on opposite walls interior to that of RF shielding. It is done to attenuate the magnetic field. It should be engineered such that minimal distortion of magnetic field occurs at the center of the scanner. Passive shielding is usually provided with the scanner.

Shimming is done to correct disturbances caused by ferromagnetic materials. The shim tolerance is provided with the scanner. For a 1.5 T magnet area where the magnetic field is equal to or greater than 5 gauss should be restricted and use should be allowed only to authorized personnel and patients who have removed all the ferromagnetic substances and are screened adequately before the scanning. Patients with implants, hearing aids, pacemakers are not suitable to undergo MR scanning High amperage power transformers, electric switchgear should be kept at a distance prescribed by the vendor with the scanner. Vibration testing of the floor has to be done so that it is minimum. Usually with departments on ground floor this problem is minimized. The room should be 30 m^2 in area. The brick and concrete construction should be adequate to absorb the acoustic noise emanating from the scanner. There should be additional space adjacent to scanner room to store the helium tank.

Helium should have access around and above the magnet. There should be space for equipment storage and centralized control of temperature and humidity factors as they affect the cryomagnetic substance and the magnetic field. Patient gurney and oxygen support inside the scanner room should be made up of MR safe materials. Warnings are to be displayed on all the entrances to indicate presence of strong magnetic field and access should be granted to authorized personnel only.

- *Ultrasound with Doppler:* Before installation of the ultrasound machine PNDT registration has to be obtained. The preconception and prenatal sex determination act (PCPNDT) keeps check on illegal sex determination of the fetus. The machine to be selected on the basis of patients to be scanned and usually it should be well equipped with a convex and linear probe, Doppler facility, Intracavitatory probe and if needed provision for 3D and 4D ultrasound. The machine should have integrated facility to store images. The prescribed form for PNDT approval then has to be filled with the required documents and then the approval is obtained. The machine can be installed only after the PNDT registration. This also needs to be periodically renewed. In cases of obstetric ultrasound consent of the patient has to be taken with completion of forms and records which are checked by the appropriate authority on inspection. It is also preferable to keep records of other general ultrasound. A board displaying the PCPNDT act and the fact that sex determination is not be done is to be displayed in English and the local language at the entrance, waiting and in the ultrasound room. Ultrasound room area should be of 25 m^2 for two machines with a partition. The ultrasound facility is to be kept away from radioactive modalities to avoid radiation hazards. There should be a separate toilet for the ultrasound patients. The room should have provisions for oxygen support and emergency drugs. If under guidance interventional procedures are done then consent of the patient is taken in writing. There should be accompanying staff nurses while doing TVS/TRS ultrasound and routinely for assistance.

- *Processing and printing room (CR):* In addition to there should be a printing and processing room near to the X-ray room of 15 m^2. This room should have the CR facility for processing and printing the digital X-ray images. PACS is to be implanted so that the acquired images are processed and stored, retrieved and presented in the DICOM format. The CR system is to accompany with a digital cassette reader and a laser printer. The system should be equipped for processing general X-rays, procedure films as well as mammography and DSA films. The CT and MR console is to be connected by local area network to the laser printer for printing of CT and MR films. There should be adequately trained technicians working in this room to ensure proper processing, printing and segregation of data according to the respective modalities.

MAINTENANCE AND MANAGEMENT

The equipment installed are to be maintained adequately for their smooth working and hence require regular technical support in the form of adequate and intelligent use and daily careful handling so that there is reduction in the usage time, and availability of credible and cost effective service with increase in the life of the instruments. In addition to this there has to be an annual maintenance contract (AMC) with adequate warranty/guarantee and emergency breakdown maintenance to be provided by the machine vendor. There should be provision for local technical support to prevent hampering of work.

Management issues are to be tackled to ensure efficient functioning of the department. Planning of infrastructure, manpower and equipment is to be done with organizing hierarchy and job responsibility distribution with maintaining a standard protocol and staff discipline. There has to be periodic evaluation to ensure adequate input is put forward to achieve favorable output in terms of quality of reporting and films with intradepartmental and patient satisfaction.

23

Molecular Imaging

Shrikant Nagare

Molecular imaging unites molecular biology and *in vivo* imaging for visualization of the cellular function and molecular process in living organisms. It has a potential for the diagnosis of diseases such as cancer, neurological and cardiovascular disorders with an aim to contribute in improving treatment. Different modalities used for noninvasive molecular imaging are, magnetic resonance imaging (MRI), optical imaging, single photon emission computed tomography (SPECT) and positron emission tomography (PET).

Visualization, characterization and measurement of biological processes at the cellular level, and going beyond to molecular levels in any living system is molecular imaging. Application of molecular imaging in clinical practice is known as molecular diagnostic imaging. Molecular imaging goes beyond structural assessment, and probes disease-specific abnormalities at the molecular level distinguishing it from classical diagnostic imaging. New genetic and molecular causes of disease are continually being discovered by means of molecular imaging. Molecular imaging has been practiced as early as 1970s in the form of using positron-emission tomography (PET) to assess blood flow in the brain and other organs using Oxygen-15 (O-15) water. Molecular imaging has only recently been defined as a separate entity. Many diseases have cellular and molecular origins, it is now recognized that imaging of processes intrinsic to metabolism may be helped by molecular imaging.

A molecular imaging system consists of a target, an agent and an imaging modality. Molecular imaging necessitates the interaction of the target with a labeled agent that can be detected externally by one or more modalities. Three major ways of agent-target interaction are recognized.

1. *Targeted binding:* The labeled agent selectively binds to its target and is detected by an external imaging modality. For example, neuroreceptor imaging in the brain with radiopharmaceutical of ^{11}C, which binds to the type-2 dopamine receptor. The interaction is detected externally by PET imaging.

2. *Imaging agent accumulation in the cell:* The structure of an agent is modified by an enzymatic action resulting in accumulation of agent in the cell. The best example is ^{18}F-fluorodeoxyglucose (FDG), which, once inside the cell, is acted upon by hexokinase, resulting in a phosphorylated version that can neither cross the cell membrane again nor undergo glycolysis. This results in the accumulation of FDG in highly metabolic cells, such as in cancer or infection/inflammation. The interaction can be detected externally by PET imaging.

3. *Activation of imaging agent by cellular components:* The imaging agent is activated by the enzymes in cell, resulting in signal amplification, e.g. bioluminescence in which the luciferase enzyme expressed by the target cell acts on injected luciferin. Emitted light is then detected externally by specialized cameras.

Prior to agent-target interaction, the imaging agent needs to be labeled. The most common labeling method is the use of modified injectable agents from known drug molecules. The *in vivo* characteristic of the labeled molecules is determined first. Favorable characteristics include, high specific activity of the label, high site selectivity and specificity; appropriate binding affinity; suitable hydro-lipophilicity and size (these features govern the transport across barriers); suitable metabolism; low immediate renal excretion, low hepatic toxicity; low nonspecific binding to reduce background signal contrast; and, the ability to achieve high local concentrations.

A limitation for the use of injectable molecular imaging agents is due to their pharmacological properties. Micro bubble ultrasound contrast agents and magnetic resonance imaging (MRI) iron nanoparticles are relatively bulky. They are restricted by body membranes like vascular endothelium, the blood-brain barrier or the cell membrane. Micro bubble ultrasound contrast agents and nanoparticles are restricted much more than low molecular weight agents.

The basis of molecular genetic imaging is indirect labeling of reporter genes. The product of a reporter gene (protein) can be detected externally. A reporter gene is genetically linked to a promoter of the gene of interest to express the gene of interest. Many new imaging agents for human reporter genes are subject to active research In anticipation of their use in human gene therapy.

Before transplantation the cells are labeled using direct cell labeling techniques. Iron oxide nanoparticles are used to label killer lymphocytes prior to reintroduction of the labeled cells into the system. These iron oxide particles provide strong negative contrast when imaged with MRI. The 3-dimensional distribution of infiltrating T-cells across the whole tumor can be detected using MRI.

MODALITIES USED FOR NONINVASIVE MOLECULAR IMAGING

Molecular imaging includes the nuclear medicine and various other fields. Nuclear medicine uses radio-labeled tracer molecules that produce signals by means of radioactive decay only. Molecular imaging uses these as well as other molecules to image via means of sound (ultrasound), magnetism magnetic resonance imaging (MRI), or light (optical techniques of bioluminescence and fluorescence) as well as other emerging techniques.

The various molecular imaging technologies differ in various aspects like spatial resolution, depth penetration and use of ionizing or nonionizing radiation, availability of injectable and biocompatible molecular markers (Fig. 23.1).

Certain imaging techniques have advantages and disadvantages over others. A variety of molecular imaging strategies are available to accomplish the increasingly sophisticated biologic interrogation of cells.

The choice of the imaging modality is determined by the temporal and spatial resolution; field of view; sensitivity of the imaging system; depth of the

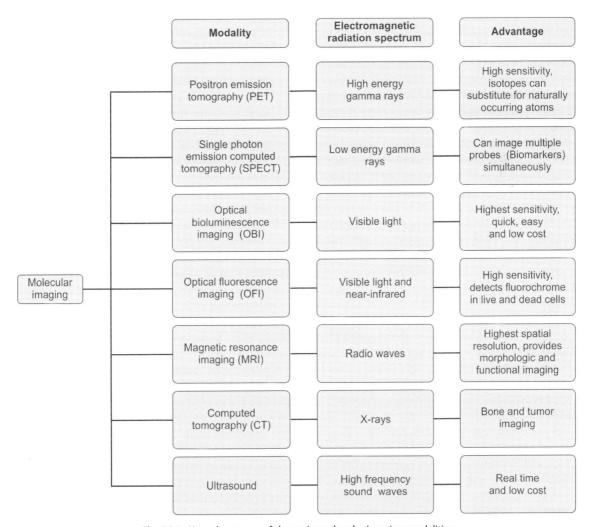

Fig. 23.1 Key advantages of the main molecular imaging modalities

biological process; the molecular or cellular process to image and the availability of suitable probes and labels that can be delivered to the imaging target.

- *Ultrasound:* Molecular imaging with ultrasound utilizes small acoustically active gas-filled micro-bubbles as specialized contrast agents. The micro-bubbles are often coated with lipids, proteins or polymers, with diameters of >1μm, which confines them to the intravascular space.

- *Optical techniques:* Optical techniques include 2 major classes: fluorescence and bioluminescence imaging. Fluorescence refers to the property of certain molecules to absorb light at a particular wavelength and to emit light of a longer wavelength after a brief interval. Photon wavelength influences the depth resolution of optical imaging techniques. Near-infrared photons currently provide the greatest wavelengths (650 nm to 900 nm) and the best depth of penetration (>1 cm).

  Bioluminescence imaging uses reporter genes that lead to expression of luciferase proteins. Upon injection of the luciferin, light is emitted as a result of a chemical reaction involving luciferase, luciferin, oxygen and ATP. The emitted light is detected externally. Optical imaging techniques are characterized by their spatial resolution varying from several millimeters to micrometer resolution and by their excellent sensitivity.

- *MRI:* MRI provides very high resolution (up to 10 μm) and unlimited depth of penetration. MRI is limited by its low sensitivity. Therefore, amplification techniques are often needed to image molecular processes. The best recognized MRI amplification technique is the use of iron oxide particles as contrast agents. These provide negative MR contrast through local increase of the relaxivity of the tissue. Superparamagnetic iron oxide (SPIO) particles are biodegradable by cellular enzymes and they provide the strongest contrast available for MR imaging. Detection is possible at micromolar concentrations of iron.

- *Nuclear medicine:* Nuclear medicine techniques provide unlimited depth penetration and have very high sensitivities. PET and single photon emission computed tomography (SPECT) cause radiation exposure and has relatively low resolution (2 mm to 5 mm for PET, 8 mm to 12 mm for SPECT). They are the most commonly used human molecular imaging modalities. PET has approximately 100 times higher sensitivity than SPECT, in large measure due to the ability to avoid using collimators during imaging. The most commonly used PET radionuclides are ^{11}C and ^{18}F. SPECT

tracers have longer half-lives, allowing the study of molecular processes that evolve over longer times. SPECT provides many readily usable radiotracers, and a local cyclotron is not needed for operation.

CLINICAL APPLICATIONS

Frequently used modalities include MRI, PET and SPECT. Optical techniques and ultrasound applications remain of limited use but they retain high potential.

Oncology

FDG is the most widely used molecular imaging agent in oncology. FDG is used as a marker of metabolism in tumor cells. FDG plays a major role in the diagnosis, evaluation and follow-up of different tumors, including lymphoma, lung cancer, brain cancer, head-and-neck tumors, melanoma, and breast cancer. FDG uptake in tumors is reflective of increased glycolysis. In brain tumors, FDG use is limited by high normal background uptake of the tracer, since the brain uses glucose as its main source of energy. This can be overcome by use of C11 methionine (MET) instead of FDG due to the lower background uptake of MET, resulting in higher tumor-to-background ratios and better visualization of the tumor.

DNA synthesis is another molecular imaging target in tumors. Thymidine kinase 1 (TK1) is an enzyme overexpressed during the DNA synthesis phase of the cell cycle. TK1 reflects cellular proliferation. ^{18}F-Fluorothymidine (FLT) is a radio labeled nucleoside analog that is phosphorylated by TK1, rendering it unable to leave the cell. FLT has been successfully used in the original evaluation as well as the follow-up and assessment of treatment response in many tumors such as lung cancer, lymphoma, head-and-neck cancer, and breast cancer.

Coated iron oxide particles are used for MRI detection of metastatic disease in lymph nodes or the liver. When injected systemically iron oxide particles are phagocytosed by macrophages and are then transported to the lymph nodes. A metastatic lymph node, in which the normal macrophage population has been replaced by tumor cells, will demonstrate partial or no drop in signal, while a normal lymph node, in which the iron particles have localized, will have decreased signal.

Inflammation and Infection

Increased FDG uptake can be seen in infectious and inflammatory conditions since FDG-PET targets the cells with relative increase in glucose metabolism in neoplastic cells over normal parenchymal cells. The main limitation of using FDG in inflammation imaging, thus, is its lack of specificity. FDG uptake of benign tumors, inflammatory processes and malignant neoplasms can sometimes overlap. To improve differentiation between neoplastic and infectious/inflammatory processes, multiple molecular imaging targets of infection/inflammation have been evaluated. Use of monoclonal antigranulocyte antibodies, such ^{99m}Tc-fanolesomab, which binds the CD15 antigen expressed on neutrophils. Radiolabeled antibiotics, on the other hand, have been used to directly target bacteria, rather than reactive cells.

Neuroimaging

Alzheimer's dementia (AD) is the most common cause of dementia. Earlier diagnosis of AD is sought for more accurate prognosis and education of the patients and their families. Several gene therapy trials are being attempted to halt or even reverse progression of AD. On FDG-PET imaging there is decreased FDG uptake in AD secondary to regional impairment of cerebral glucose metabolism in neocortical association areas. Primary visual areas, the sensorimotor cortex, basal ganglia, and cerebellum are relatively well preserved. FDG-PET abnormalities however are not pathognomonic of AD. Alternative molecular imaging targets are sought for higher specificity. The most intuitive targets are the pathologic associates of AD, namely neurofibrillary tangles (NFTs) and amyloid plaques (APs). Novel PET and SPECT ligands for NFTs and APs are under investigation. The best known amyloid ligand currently is the ^{11}C-labeled Pittsburgh compound B (PIB). AD patients show increased retention of PIB in association cortex areas known to contain large amounts of amyloid deposits in AD, compared with controls. However, cognitively normal controls with higher than normal PIB uptake were noted, raising the possibility of those subjects being predisposed to develop AD.

24

Nuclear Medicine Physics

Sujit Nilagaonkar

BASIC ATOMIC AND NUCLEAR PHYSICS

The atom is considered to be the basic building block of all matter. It represents the physical and chemical characteristics of that material. It consists of two components: a nucleus and orbiting electrons which surround the nucleus. The nucleus is said to be positively charged and the electrons negatively charged. The nuclei are composed of protons and neutrons, collectively called nucleons. Protons are positively charge, neutrons are electrically neutral and orbiting electrons are negatively charged.

Notation of an atom:

$$_Z^A X_N$$

Where, A - is atomic mass number (Z + N), X- is the element, Z - Atomic number (i.e. number of protons) and N- is number of neutrons.

Isotopes: Isotopes are the radionuclides with the same number of protons (z). These are the same elements but with different number of neutrons. e.g. I^{123}, I^{125}, I^{131}.

In classical Bohr's model of atom, the electrons are described as arranged in well-defined orbits around the nucleus. Electrons are basic elementary particles. Orbital electrons are the electrons in orbits in an atom. Orbital electrons in each atom are equal to the number of protons in the nucleus. The closest orbit to the nucleus is referred as K-shell and next one is referred to as L, M and N so forth. The maximum number of electrons in the K-shell is 2 and in the L shell is 8, in M shell is 18 and in N-shell is 32. Outer most orbit cannot have more than 8 electrons. Valence electrons are the electrons in the outermost shell of an atom. These electrons are responsible for defining the chemical properties of the element.

RADIOACTIVE DECAY

The term radioactivity refers to the emission of particles and/or energy from unstable isotopes. Because of physical properties, certain atoms are unstable and radioactive decay is a process used by unstable atoms to achieve a more stable situation.

The term X-ray is used for the emission of photons from outside the nucleus and gamma ray is used for photons originating in the nucleus.

From nuclear medicine point of view; gamma rays, beta particles, positrons and alpha particles are important.

Methods of Radioactive Decay

Alpha Decay

Alpha decay is common in the higher atomic number range of the periodic table.

In this decay process alpha particles are essentially helium nuclei with a +2 charge and an atomic mass number of 4.

Alpha particles are undesirable in diagnostic application, but favorable therapeutic agents have been designed.

e.g. Uranium^{238} nucleus.

$$_{92}^{238}U \rightarrow _{90}^{234}U + _2^4He$$

The uranium-238 nucleus emits a helium-4 nucleus (the alpha particle) and the parent nucleus becomes thorium-234.

Beta Decay

Beta decay is also called as negatron decay. There are three common forms of beta decay. In beta decay the conversion of a neutron into a proton, an electron and a subatomic particle called antineutrino. The electron is ejected from the atomic nucleus.

Gamma Decay

Gamma decay involves the emission of energy from an unstable nucleus in the form of electromagnetic radiation. Gamma rays are emitted almost immediately after the primary decay process whether it is alpha decay, negatron decay.

The radioactive decay equation and half-life concept: The decay process is dependent upon the initial

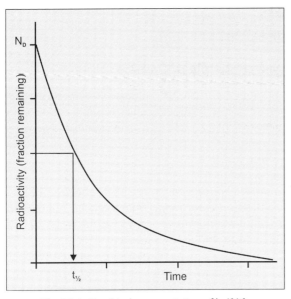

Fig. 24.1 Graphical representation of half-life

number of nuclei present, i.e. N and on the time period. Suppose initial number of nuclei is N at time T0. Let us assume that dN is the number of nuclei decayed over a period dT.

Half-life: It is the time required for a radionuclide to decay to 50% of the initial activity level. Note that the half-life does not express how long a material will remain radioactive but simply the length of time for its radioactivity to halve of initial activity (Fig. 24.1).

Biological half-life: This term is used to describe biological clearance of a radionuclide from a particular tissue or organ. The term biological half-life is useful in anticipating about the amount of exposure the patient actually receives during a nuclear medicine procedure.

Effective half-life: It is the actual half-life of a radiopharmaceutical in a biological system.

It is dependent on both the physical half-life and biological half-life.

Units of Radioactivity

The SI or metric unit of radioactivity is named after Henri Becquerel, in honor of his discovery of radioactivity, and is called the Becquerel with the symbol "Bq".

The Becquerel is defined as the quantity of radioactive substance that gives rise to a decay rate of 1 decay per second (1dps).

The traditional unit of radioactivity is named after Marie Curie and is called the curie, with the symbol Ci.

The curie is defined as the amount of radioactive substance which gives rise to a decay rate of

$$3.7 \times 10^{10} \text{ decays per second.}$$

Interaction of Radiation with Matter

During radioactive decay, two types of radiation are emitted.
a. Charged particles such as alpha particles and beta particles
b. Electromagnetic radiation such as gamma rays and X-rays.

These radiations transfer their energy to the matter by ionization and excitation of atoms and molecules as they pass through it.

The charged particles when passed through matter cause ionization by transforming energy to the matter, therefore, they are important for radiation dosimetry as well.

RADIATION DETECTORS

Basic Principle

When a photon strikes a detector material, it causes ionization and excitation by photoelectric and Compton scatter methods. When the ionized atoms undergo de-excitation, energy is released. Most of the energy is released as thermal energy, but some energy is released as visible light.

Scintillators: These are the materials which produce visible light after interaction of photons with the matter. And the detectors made from such scintillators are called scintillation detectors.

There are two types of detector materials one is detectors made up of organic substances and other are detectors made up of inorganic substances.

Photomultiplier Tubes

Photomultiplier tube (PMT) is an electronic device which produces a pulse of electric current when stimulated by weak light signal and multiplies it to several folds thus converting a relatively small light signal into a large pulse of current. PMTs are available in various size and shapes like round, hexagonal, square, etc. PMT is basically tubes sealed in glass and evacuated tubes wrapped in metal foil for magnetic shielding. PMTs are maintained at high voltage levels. PMTs made up of multiple dynodes which are maintained at higher voltage levels than another (Fig. 24.2). The PMT has a glass entrance window. The surface of the glass window is covered by a photo emissive substance. This photo emissive surface is called photocathode. When the photo emissive surface is struck by visible light, it emits electrons. These electrons are called photoelectrons. Focusing grid is

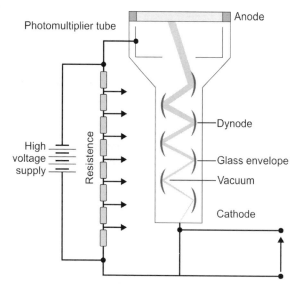

Fig. 24.2 Basic structure and working photomultiplier tube

placed between dynodes and photo emissive surface. This grid directs the photoelectrons towards dynodes.

Inorganic Scintillators

These are the solid state materials which scintillate in crystal form. The most commonly used scintillator in nuclear medicine is NaI (Tl) crystal. The crystal is doped with Thallium impurity to make them operable at room temperature.

Characteristics of NaI (Tl) Crystal

Advantages

- It is relatively dense and with high atomic number—therefore it is good absorber and efficient detector.
- It gives good light output—i.e. efficient scintillators producing one visible light photon per 30 eV of radiation.
- It is transparent to its own radiation-therefore little loss of scintillation light.
- Crystals of large size can be grown in ovens at relatively small costs.
- Wavelength well matched to peak response to PMT.

Disadvantages

- Fragile and easily fracturable crystal
- Hygroscopic in nature—if absorbs moisture, light transmission from detector to PMT is hampered.
- For higher energy gamma rays detection, larger volumes of detector are required.

NUCLEAR MEDICINE IMAGING SYSTEM

Basic Principle of Gamma Camera

Components of gamma camera are collimator, NaI (Tl) crystal, photomultiplier tube, position logic circuit, pulse height analyzer and display monitor.

Collimator

Gamma rays cannot be focused. The gamma rays originating from the patient must be focused on the camera system to form an image. In nuclear medicine, patient itself is a source of gamma rays. The rays coming out from the patient are distributed in all directions.

This includes gamma rays which are having significant clinical information and those gamma rays which are distorted and do not travel in expected direction.

Therefore, it is necessary to prevent gamma rays which are not traveling in proper direction.

Collimators, here play role of absorptive collimation by absorbing the unwanted gamma rays before they reach detector. The image is produced by allowing only those rays which are traveling in certain direction to reach detector.

Collimators are formed of metals having high density and high atomic number. Lead with atomic number 82 and density 11.3 g/cm cube is most commonly used for collimator.

Holes are drilled in lead. The lead walls between the septa are called collimator septa. The septal thickness, diameter of hole and length of septa are characteristics for a particular collimator.

Detector System and Electronics

The gamma camera is formed by a large NaI (Tl) detector crystal, usually 6 mm to 12 mm thickness and 35 to 50 cm in diameter. Because of hygroscopic nature of the crystal material, the detector crystal is completely sealed with thin aluminum casing. The front surface of crystal is surrounded by a highly reflective material TiO_2 to maximize light output. An optical glass window is kept on back surface of the casing for permitting the scintillation light to reach the PM tube. All detector electronics such as preamplifier, pulse height analyzer, automatic gain control and pulse pileup rejection circuits are directly employed on the individual PM tube bases.

Event Analysis and Positioning

When an event occurs and it is analyzed by pulse height analyzer. If it falls within the acceptable energy window, the event is labeled as X and Y co-ordinates and it is binned in pixels. Each pixel should have sufficient number of counts detected so as to form an interpretable image.

In modern gamma cameras, the output from a PMT is directly digitalized by analog to digital converter and the event position is calculated in software.

Only those gamma rays whose energy fall within acceptable energy window 130 Kev to 150 Kev are selected for the counting. Therefore energy selection becomes important to improve image resolution.

PRODUCTION OF RADIOISOTOPES

Most of the radioisotopes found in nature have relatively long half-lives. As a result medical applications generally require the use of radioisotopes which are produced artificially.

A stable nucleus is converted into an unstable nucleus by bombarding the nuclei by protons or neutrons.

The Production Methods

- Reactor produced: Nuclear reactors have been a source of radioisotope production since a long period of time.

    The production mainly takes place by
    - Nuclear fission
    - Nuclear bombardment
- Accelerator produced:
    - Positive ion cyclotron
    - Negative ion cyclotron

Radioisotope Generator

Radioisotope generator consists of a relatively long-lived radioisotope (parent) which decays into the short-lived isotope of interest (daughter). A good example is ^{99m}Tc which is the most widely used radioisotope in nuclear medicine today. The ^{99}Mo is called the parent isotope. This isotope has a half-life of six hours.

The chemical separation device is called, in this example, a ^{99m}Tc Generator. Column Generator System consists of a ceramic column with ^{99}Mo adsorbed onto its top surface (Fig. 24.3). A solution called an eluent is passed through the column, reacts chemically with any ^{99m}Tc and emerges in a chemical form which is suitable for combining with a pharmaceutical to produce a radiopharmaceutical. The ceramic column and collection vials need to be surrounded

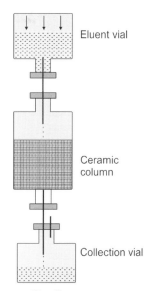

Fig. 24.3 Mo^{99}- Tc^{99m} column generator system

by lead shielding for radiation protection purposes. In addition all components are produced and need to be maintained in a sterile condition.

CYCLOTRON

A cyclotron (Fig. 24.4) is a type of charged particle accelerator in which electrically charged subnuclear particles as protons, deuterons and alpha particles accelerate outwards from the center along a spiral path. The particles are held to a spiral trajectory by a static magnetic field and accelerated by a rapidly varying (radio frequency) electric field. The energy of the particle increases as the velocity of the particle increases. The cyclotron utilizes this fact to produce particles of reasonably high energy in a relatively confined space. When the accelerated beam reaches its maximum energy it can be directed onto a target material causing nuclear reactions to occur that result in the formation of radionuclides.

Cyclotrons were the best source of high-energy beams for nuclear physics experiments in past. Cyclotrons can be used in particle therapy to treat cancer. Ion beams from cyclotrons can be used, as in proton therapy, to penetrate the body and kill tumors by radiation damage, while minimizing damage to healthy tissue along their path. Cyclotron beams can be used to bombard other atoms to produce short-lived positron-emitting isotopes (18FDG glucose) suitable for PET imaging.

TECHNETIUM-99M

Technetium-99m is a metastable radioactive tracer which emits gamma rays from within the body to

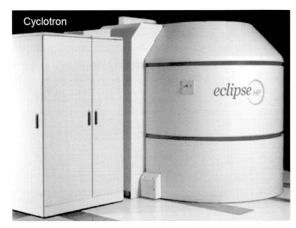

Fig. 24.4 Cyclotron

provide information about the functioning of a person's specific organs, symbolized as ^{99m}Tc. It is the most commonly-used medical radioisotope.

Technetium-99m when used as a radioactive tracer can be detected in the body by gamma cameras. It is well suited to the role because it emits readily detectable 140 keV gamma rays which are about the same wavelength as emitted by conventional X-ray diagnostic equipment. The half-life for gamma emission is about 6.0058 hours. The "short" physical half-life and its biological half-life of 1 day allows rapid data collection, but keep total patient radiation exposure low. The same characteristics make the isotope suitable only for diagnostic but never therapeutic use. Molybdenum-99 is used commercially as the easily-transportable source of medically used Tc-99m.

It is used for imaging and functional studies of the brain, myocardium, thyroid, lungs, liver, gallbladder, kidneys, skeleton, blood, and tumors.

Diagnostic treatment involving technetium-99m will result in radiation exposure to technicians, patients, and passers-by. The doses used in scintigraphy result in radiation exposures to the patient around 10 mSv, the equivalent of about 500 chests X-ray exposures. This level of radiation exposure carries a 1 in 1000 lifetime risk of developing a solid cancer or leukemia in the patient. The risk is higher in younger patients, and lower in older ones. The radiation source is inside the patient and will be carried around for a few days, exposing others to second-hand radiation.

RADIONUCLIDE SCANNING

Lungs

Radionuclide scanning of the lungs is performed for detection of pulmonary embolism, preoperative evaluation of regional pulmonary function, detection of venous thrombosis and fat embolism.

Radionuclides Used for Scanning of Lungs

Perfusion agent are ^{99m}Technetium -MAA (macro aggregated albumin) and ^{99m}Technetium (human albumin microspheres).

Ventilation agents are ^{133}Xenon and ^{99m}Technetium –DTPA (diethylene triamine pentaacetic acid).

Various Techniques for Isotope Imaging of Lung

Radioactive gases
- ^{133}Xe: Ventilation studies with Xe-133 are ordinarily performed first during combined V/Q imaging. A large field of view gamma camera with a low energy all purpose collimator is used. The usual adult dose of Xe-133 is 10 to 20 mCi. The patient is seated (if possible) with the camera positioned in the posterior view.
- *First breath:* The patient exhales fully and is asked to take a maximal inspiration and hold it long enough, if possible, to obtain 100k counts.
- *Equilibrium:* Obtain two sequential 45 sec poster images while the patient breathes normally.
- *Washout:* Obtain three sequential 45 sec posterior images and then left and right posterior oblique images and a final posterior image.

Radio aerosols: For studies with radio aerosols the radiopharmaceutical is placed in a special nebulizer system. The patient is asked to breathe through the mouth piece of the delivery system until sufficient radio aerosol is delivered to the lungs. 25 to 30 mCi of ^{99m}Tc -DTPA (diethylene triamine pentaacetic acid) is used. The views obtained in radio aerosol studies should be the same as those obtained for the perfusion phase in anterior, posterior, right and left lateral and both posterior 45 degree oblique views. ^{99m}Tc-DTPA aerosols remain in the lung, with a biological half-life approaching 1 hour.

Perfusion imaging: ^{99m}Tc MAA, 4 mCi adult dose is injected intravenously over several respiratory cycles with the patient in supine position. A large field of view gamma camera with a low energy high resolution or all purpose collimator and a 20% window centered at 140 Kev is used. The views obtained phase in anterior, posterior, right and left lateral and both posterior 45° oblique views. The right and left 45° anterior oblique views. Obtain 500 k to 750 k counts per image.

Clinical Implication

- *Ventilation perfusion mismatch:* Abnormal perfusion in an area of normal ventilation or much larger perfusion abnormality than ventilation defect.

- *Ventilation perfusion match:* Both scintigrams are abnormal in the same area: defects of equal size.
- *Segmental defect:* Caused by occlusion of a branch of the pulmonary artery, typical wedge shaped and pleural based. Conforms to segmental anatomy of lung.

Diagnostic Criteria

The multi institutional modified PIOPED (Prospective Investigation of Pulmonary Embolism Diagnosis) criteria for combined study interpretation:
- High probability (80–100%)
- Intermediate probability (20–80%)
- Low probability (<20%)
- Normal study.

For high probability criteria, the likely hood of pulmonary embolism is >80%. The hallmark is a perfusion defect corresponding to a broncho-pulmonary segment with normal ventilation and normal chest radiograph.

When the perfusion study is completely normal without a segmental defect, the likelihood of PE is less than 5%. The likelyhood of significant morbidity or mortality from PE is probably less than 1%.

Hepatobiliary Scanning

Radioisotopes used in hepatobiliary scanning are analogs of ^{99m}Tc IDA (Iminodiacetic acid)
- *HIDA:* Hydroxy iminodiacetic acid
  85% excreted by the liver, 15% by the kidneys
  Good visualization at bilirubin levels of 5–7 mg/dL
- Disofenin (Mebrofenin)
  It has greatest resistance to displacement by bilirubin. Over 80% of the administered activity is cleared from the blood by liver hepatocytes within 10 minutes.
  Half-life (T1/2) of uptake is about 6 minutes, and the T1/2 of excretion is about 14 minutes.

Technique

Standard Examination

The patient should be fasting for 4 to 8 hrs; Narcotics that act on the sphincter of Oddi should be stopped 6 to 12 hours prior to the examination.

Normal examination reveals the liver activity exceeds cardiac blood pool by 5 minutes and by 10 minutes the cardiac blood pool activity gets diminished. Persistent blood pool activity indicates hepatocellular dysfunction. Biliary activity is typically seen by 15 minutes and over 90% of normal studies the gallbladder is visualized within 30 minutes. About 80% of normal patients small bowel activity is visualized within 60 minutes and most of the patients show it within 90 minutes. If activity is seen within the gallbladder, but not in the small bowel by 90 minutes of the study, Sincalide may be used to expedite small bowel visualization and measure gallbladder ejection fraction.

Cholecystokinin in Hepatobiliary Imaging

Cholecystokinin (CCK) is released endogenously by the duodenal mucosa in response to a fatty meal. Gallbladder contraction is initiated when the serum CCK concentration reaches a threshold. CCK also acts to relax the sphincter of Oddi allowing bile to empty into the small bowel.

Sincalide (synthetic CCK) reproduces the active portion of CCK, the C-terminal octapeptide fragment. The most commonly administered dose is 0.02 ug/kg given by slow I.V. infusion typically over 4 to 5 minutes, Gallbladder contraction begins rapidly following sincalide infusion, with a maximal effect within 15 minutes.

Indications for the use of Sincalide include patient fasting for more than 20 to 24 hours and the determination of gall bladder ejection fraction (GBEF).

Morphine Augmented Cholescintigraphy

Morphine can be used to decrease the time required to confirm acute cholecystitis. Dose: 0.04 mg/kg (Max. 2–3 mg) given over a 3 minute infusion. Morphine may be administered after 45 minutes to 1 hour if the gallbladder is not visualized, and there is:
- No evidence of CBD obstruction, and
- Sufficient activity remains within the liver to allow for subsequent imaging.

Morphine can produce up to a 10 fold increase in the resting pressure of the common bile duct by causing contraction of the sphincter of Oddi.

If GB has not filled by 30 minutesafter morphine injection the exam is diagnostic of acute cholecystitis. Visualization of the gallbladder 5 to 30 minutes after morphine is indicative of chronic cholecystitis. Overall, the sensitivity (96 to 100%) and specificity (81 to 100%).

Indications

- Cholecystitis
- Bile leak
- Biliary dyskinesia
- Hepatic arterial perfusion scintigraphy
- Biliary atresia
- Neonatal hepatitis
- Choledocal cyst.

Renal Scanning

In renal scan different agents are used for assessing various parameters of renal functions.

Agents used to quantify glomerular function is ^{99m}Technetium DTPA.

Agents used to quantify effective renal plasma flow are ^{131}I orthoidohippurate and ^{99m}Technetium mercaptoacetyltriglycine.

Agents used for renal cortical scintigraphy are ^{99m}Tc DMSA (Dimercaptosuccinic acid) and ^{99m}Tc gluco heptonate (GHA).

Techniques

Quantitative evaluation of clearance
- Under steady state conditions
  - Constant infusion method
  - Feedback controlled infusion method
- During slope (single injection)
  - Multiple blood sampling
    - Two compartment model
    - Single compartment model
    - Stewart-Hamilton principle
  - Single sample method
  - External counting method
    - Diuretic renography.

Indications of Renography

- Obstructive uropathy
  Clinical applications
  - Need of intervention—in cases of equivocal obstruction diagnosis the intervention decision depends upon presence or absence of obstruction and relative function of the kidney.
    Renography contributed to decision making process how to intervene
  - Type of intervention—by determination of split function, relative function of each kidney can be determined. This helps surgeons to decide up to what extent function must be preserved.
    In cases of obstructive kidney, it helps surgeons to determine the amount of recoverable function
- Idiopathic hydronephrosis
  Clinical application—In conditions in which dilatation is apparent but no cause is demonstrated, the key to management is distinguishing between stasis and obstruction. Diuretic renography plays important role in decision making.

- Primary megaureter
  Clinical application
  - To exclude refluxing or nonrefluxing system obstructive or nonobstructive excretory system.
  - Postsurgery to see the success of surgery and to pick up postoperative complication.
    For example, stenosis at vesicouretic junction.
  - In cases where conservative approach is used renography is used to monitor progress.
- Urinary calculi
  - Acute obstruction—diagnosed by IVU and USG
    Clinical implication of renography-
    - Gives information regarding function of the kidneys
    - Gives information regarding degree of obstruction and reduction in ipsilateral function which helps to decide urgency of intervention and provides a baseline
  - Monitoring of progress
    Clinical implication
    - Need of accurate and reliable means of measuring and monitoring progress
    - To monitor increasing obstruction or deterioration of split function which needs intervention.
  - Bilateral calculus disease:
    Clinical implication: Split renal function analysis may influence the decision regarding the type and timing of operation.
    - In deciding which kidney to operate first.
  - Borderline function
    Clinical implication: The management decision depends between removing the calculus or performing a nephrectomy.
    - Relative function measurement is essential in decision making.
    - Repeat scan after nephrostomy may be necessary to determine the amount of recoverable function before a final decision is made.
- Renal transplant evaluation
- VUR—Methods
  - Direct radionuclide cystogram
  - Indirect radionuclide cystogram
    Advantages: High sensitivity, low radiation burden to the child
- Renovascular hypertension evaluation.

Indications of Renal Cortical Imaging Agents

- To detect focal areas of renal parenchymal defects
- Acute pyelonephritis

- Renovascular disease
- To evaluate renal scars
- Complex duplex systems
- Ectopic kidney evaluation
- Evaluation of poorly functioning kidneys.

RADIONUCLIDE AGENTS USED IN NEUROIMAGING

- Conventional brain scintigraphy
  - ^{99m}Tc- glucoheptonate (GH)
  - ^{99m}Tc-diethylene-triamine-pentaacetic acid (DTPA)
- Brain perfusion scintigraphy
  - ^{123}I iodoamphetamine (IMP)
  - ^{99m}Tc Tc-Hexamethylpropyleneamine Oxime (HMPAO)
  - ^{99m}Tc- methyl cycteinate dimer (ECD)
- Brian tumor imaging
  - ^{201}Thallium
  - ^{99m}Tc sestamibi
- Cisternography
  - ^{111}Indium –DTPA
- Positron emission tomography

Compound	Application
^{18}Flurine -fluorodeoxy-glucose	glucose utilization
^{15}Oxygen O_2	oxygen metabolism
^{15}Oxygen H_2O	blood flow
^{11}Carbon methionine	amino acid metabolism
^{11}Carbon methylspiperone	dopamine receptor activity
^{11}Carbon carfentanil	opiate receptor activity
^{11}Carbon flunitrazepam	benzodiazepine receptor activity
^{11}Carbon scopolamine	muscarinic cholinergic receptor
^{18}Flurine fluoro-L-DOPA	Presynaptic dopaminergic system
^{11}Carbon ephedrine	adrenergic terminals
^{11}Carbon or ^{15}Oxygen carboxyhemoglobin	blood volume

Conventional Brain Scintigraphy

Diseases of the brain cause a breakdown in the blood brain barrier which permits the uptake of conventional brain imaging agents. Other than for brain death, conventional brain scintigraphy is no longer routinely performed.

SPECT Brain Perfusion Scintigraphy

Brain SPECT imaging provides complementary functional information to anatomic imaging exams. SPECT agents such as Tc-HMPAO and Tc-ECD reflect cerebral perfusion.

Brain SPECT Imaging in Dementia

Dementias produce deficits in perfusion, in part reflecting decreased metabolic needs. Characteristic patterns have a predictive value of over 80% for the diagnosis of Alzheimer's disease. A correlation has also been described between the severity of these defects, and the severity of the patient's dementia.

Brain SPECT in Psychiatric Disorders

Tc99m-HMPAO may be more useful than EEG in determining response to therapy in patients with psychiatric disorders.

Brain SPECT for the Detection of a Seizure Focus

Epilepsy is one of the most prevalent neurological disorders—affecting about 1% of the general population. The most common pathologic finding in these patients is mesial temporal sclerosis which is thought to represent a gliotic scar. Excision of this focus can lead to elimination of the seizures or significantly improved pharmacologic control in 80% of patients. CT and MRI have low sensitivity for seizure foci detection, 17% and 34% respectively. The role of brain SPECT is to localize the seizure focus.

The ictal exam requires that the patient be placed in a special room with continuous video and EEG monitoring. The patients medication is usually tapered off or discontinued to increase the likelihood of a seizure episode. The tracer to be injected at the time of ictal phase and imaging is done after 40 minutes of injection. Inter ictal study is conducted and both images sets are compared to localize seizure focus.

CNS Vascular Imaging

Tc99m-cerebral perfusion studies can be used to confirm the presence of cerebral infarction, monitor the effects of acute thrombolytic therapy and to predict stroke outcome.

CSF Flow Studies

CSF flow studies are performed using either In-111 (DTPA) or Tc99mDTPA. Indications for the exam include suspected normal pressure hydrocephalus, occult CSF rhinorrhea/otorrhea and ventricular shunt evaluation.

Brain Tumors

Viable areas within CNS neoplasms are generally expected to demonstrate increased metabolism, while areas of necrosis show no metabolic activity.

25
Miscellaneous

Hariqbal Singh

RESISTORS

A **resistor** is two-terminal electrical component that implements electrical resistance as a circuit element. The current through a resistor is in direct proportion to the voltage across the resistor's terminals. Ohm's law states the ratio of the voltage applied across a resistor's terminals to the intensity of current through the circuit is proportional to resistance.

$$I = V/R$$

Where, I is the current through the conductor in units of amperes.

V is the potential difference measured across the conductor in units of volts.

R is the resistance of the conductor in units of Ohms.

Series and Parallel Resistors

A series circuit (Fig. 25.1) is a circuit in which resistors are arranged in a chain, so the current has only one path to take. The current is the same through each resistor. The total resistance of the circuit is found by simply adding up the resistance values of the individual resistors.

Equivalent resistance of resistors in series: $R = R_1 + R_2 + R_3 + ... R_n$

A parallel circuit (Fig. 25.2) is a circuit in which the resistors are arranged in parallel. The current in a parallel circuit breaks up, with some flowing along each parallel branch and re-combining when the branches meet again. The voltage across each resistor in parallel is the same. The total resistance of a set of resistors in parallel is found by adding up the reciprocals of the resistance values and then taking the reciprocal of the total. Equivalent resistance of resistors in parallel: $1/R = 1/R_1 + 1/R_2 + 1/R_3 + ... 1/R_n$

ATTENUATION AND ABSORPTION

Attenuation is the reduction of the intensity of an X-ray beam as it traverses matter. The reduction may be caused by absorption or deflection of photons from the beam (scatter).

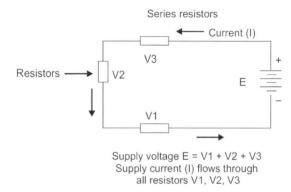

Supply voltage E = V1 + V2 + V3
Supply current (I) flows through all resistors V1, V2, V3

Fig. 25.1 Resistors in series

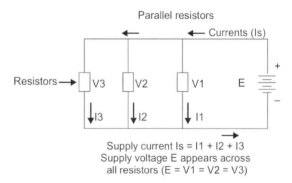

Supply current Is = I1 + I2 + I3
Supply voltage E appears across all resistors (E = V1 = V2 = V3)

Fig. 25.2 Resistors in parallel

Attenuation = Absorption + Scatter

Absorption: X-rays are said to be absorbed when they transfer all or part of their energy to the matter. The photoelectric effect is the predominant interaction with low energy radiation and with high atomic number absorbers. It generates no significant scatter radiation and produces high contrast in the X-ray image but, unfortunately, exposes the patient to a great deal of radiation.

TUBE RATING CHARTS

With careful use, the X-ray tube can provide long periods of service. Inconsiderate or careless operation can lead to shortened life or abrupt failure. Tube life is extended by use of minimum mAs and kVp appropriate for the examination. Manufacturers combine heat loading characteristics and information about the limits of their X-ray tubes in graphical representations called Tube Rating Charts. Use of faster image receptor requires lower mAs and kVp which extends tube life. It is essential for the X-ray operator to understand how to use tube rating charts.

A procedure generates an amount of heat depending on: kV used, tube current (mA), length of exposure, type of voltage waveform and number of exposures taken in rapid sequence.

Thermal energy in X-ray is measured in Heat Units (HU)

Heat Unit (HU) [joule]: Unit of potential x unit of tube current x unit of time

There are three types of charts.

1. Radiographic Rating Charts

A tube may be used in many ways with many variables. Even the angle of the anode is important. Always look at the correct chart. The x-axis and y-axis are graduated in kVp and time respectively. The mA is graphed as a curved line. Any combination of kVp and Time below the line should be safe for a single exposure.

2. Anode Cooling Chart

Heat generated is stored in the anode and dissipated through the cooling circuit. A typical cooling chart has input curves (heat units stored as a function of time) and anode cooling curve. The anode has a limited capacity for storing heat. Heat is continuously dissipated to the oil bath and tube housing by conduction and radiation. It is possible through prolonged use of multiple exposures to exceed the heat storage capacity of the anode. This chart is not dependent upon the filament size or speed of anode rotation. The cooling is rapid at first but slows as the anode cools. It is not uncommon for it to take 15 minutes to cool the tube.

3. Housing Cooling Charts

The tube housing cooling chart is very similar to the anode cooling chart. The tube housing will generally have a capacity of about 1 to 1.5 million HU. Complete cooling may take 1 to 2 hours.

The capacity of the focal spot track is generally specified by the manufacturer in the form of a graph or tube rating chart. Curved lines show the maximum power (KV and MA) that can be delivered to the tube for a given exposure. From these graphs we see that the safe power limit is inversely related to the exposure time. Remember that the total heat delivered to the tube is the product of the power and exposure

time. Therefore it is not only the total amount of heat delivered to the tube that is crucial, but also the time in which it is delivered.

THE INVERSE SQUARE LAW

The inverse square law applies to any entity which radiates out from a point in space. An inverse-square law is any *physical law* stating that a specified physical *quantity* or strength is *inversely proportional* to the *square* of the *distance* from the source of that physical quantity. Since the initial beam travels in straight but divergent directions, geometry in a three dimensional world dictates that the radiation intensity will decrease with the inverse square of the distance. Consequently, the number of X-rays traveling through a unit area decreases with increasing distance. Likewise, radiation level decreases with increasing distance since exposure is directly proportional to the number of X-rays interacting in a unit area. In other words the strength of the X-ray beam is inversely proportional to the square of distance from the source. Standing back by double the distance from a source of radiation will quarter the dose to the radiologist or radiographer. The intensity of the radiation is described by the inverse square law equation:

$$X_A \propto X_B \left[\frac{DA}{DB}\right]^2$$

Where X_A is the radiation exposure rate at distance DA compared with the exposure rate X_B at some other distance D_B.

DARKROOM

A darkroom is a room that is completely dark to allow the processing of light sensitive photographic material like photographic film. It is a place where the necessary handling and processing of film can be carried out safely and efficiently without hazard of producing film fog by accidental exposure to light or X-ray. Darkrooms contain film processors, a loading bench, a film bin for storage of unexposed radiographic film, a film ID printer, safelights and a pass box in the wall which allows transfer of film/cassettes to and from the darkroom, while ensuring no light is admitted to the darkroom.

Convenient placement of darkroom saves time and eliminates unnecessary steps. It should be readily accessible to plumbing and electrical services. Lead shielding is essential if adjacent to X-ray room. 1/16 inch of lead in the walls all the way to the ceiling. Passboxes should be built at appropriate location and have two light tight and X-ray proof interlocked doors. Walls should be covered with chemical resistant material. Walls of the darkroom are painted a light color to help reflect the safelights.

The darkroom and all the equipment and accessories should be kept spotless. Noxious fumes may present with use of today's auto processors. Therefore, ventilation near the processor is needed. Make sure that the ventilation system is lightproof. Three type of entrance are known, interlocked two doors, maze type and revolving door. A safelight is the room light that will not fog photographic materials during the time period required for normal handling and processing. It provides illumination only from parts of the visible spectrum to which the photographic material in use is nearly or completely insensitive. The word "safe" in «safelight» is relative, as in most cases a sensitized material will eventually be affected by its safelight if exposed to it for an extended length of time. A source of overhead light is essential for general purposes like cleaning, changing solution. A warning light should be located outside the darkroom, at the entrance, to indicate when the room is in use.

Films must be handled with clean, dry hands, and touched only at the corners. Dirt or chemical residue on hand can cause unwanted marks on the film or may stain the intensifying screens on the cassettes. Cassettes should be reloaded as soon as possible after unloading, to prevent dirt from getting into the cassette. Cassettes that have been exposed to radiation must be kept separate from cassettes loaded with unexposed film to avoid the possibility of accidentally reusing an exposed cassette.

The major equipment in darkroom is manual processing tanks and film hangers. The conventional darkroom has become outdated followed by automatic film processors, which has also become out of vogue. Most medical imaging departments to day use computed radiography or digital radiography which does not require any darkroom.

SAFE LIGHT

A safelight is a light illumination suitable for use in a photographic darkroom that will not fog photographic materials during the time period required for normal handling and processing. It provides illumination only from parts of the visible spectrum to which the photographic material in use is nearly or completely insensitive.

A safelight usually consists of an ordinary light bulb in a housing closed off by a colored filter, but sometimes a special light bulb or fluorescent tube with suitable filter material coated directly on the glass is used in an ordinary fixture. Differently sensitized materials require different safelights. In traditional black-and-white photographic printing, photographic papers are normally handled under amber or red safelight; as such papers are typically sensitive only to blue and green light. Different filters are available for orthochromatic, panchromatic films. The working distance should be more than one meter. The bulb wattage should correspond to that specified on the lamp housing.

The safety of darkroom lighting may be tested as follows: Subject a film in cassette to a very small exposure, just enough to cause slight graying. Then remove the film from cassette in the darkroom, cover one half of the film with black paper and leave it exposed under conditions simulating as closely as possible those normally existing when a film is being loaded and unloaded. Process the film as usual. If the uncovered portion appears darker than covered, conclude that safelight is unsafe.

NEGATIVE CONTRAST AGENTS

Contrast media are so called as they increase the image contrast of anatomical structures which are not normally easily visualized. The negative radiological contrast media are the gases air, oxygen, nitric oxide (N_2O) or carbon dioxide (CO_2). They may be combined with water suspensions of barium sulfate for double contrast images of the gastrointestinal tract and with water soluble iodinated contrast media for double contrast investigations of joints. Air can be used as a contrast material because it is less radiopaque than the tissues it is defining.

Examples of the use of negative contrast medium are Double Contrast Barium Enema, Double Contrast Barium Meal, CT Pneumocolon/Virtual Colonoscopy, the use of air bubbles to aid the sonographic detection.

The use of gas as a contrast medium in the gastrointestinal tract has no other adverse effects than those induced by the volume of the gas.

Gas emboli may occur from unintentional intravascular injection of gas. The danger of injecting gas decreases with smaller gas volumes and higher water solubility of the injected gas. Carbon dioxide has the highest water solubility and there is an increased interest in using carbon dioxide in for example, femoral arteriography because the digital subtraction technique may produce images of workable quality. An advantage is of course the low price of the gas. Gas may only be used in areas that the examiner considers will tolerate a transient reduction or transient interruption of blood flow.

LINEAR TOMOGRAPHY

Tomography is the imaging modality in which only structures in a selected plane of the patient, parallel to the film, are imaged sharply and everything else above and below appears blurred to the point they become unrecognisable.

In linear tomography the movement is along linear path. The essential ingredients are an X-ray tube, an X-ray film and a rigid connecting rod that rotates about a fixed fulcrum. When the tube moves in one direction, the film moves in the opposite direction. The film is placed in a tray under the X-ray table so that it is free to move without disturbing the patient. The fulcrum is the only point in the system that remains stationary. The amplitude of tube travel is measured in degrees, and is called the tomographic angle (arc). The plane of interest within the patient is positioned at the level of the fulcrum and it is the only plane that remains in sharp focus. All points above and below this plane are blurred.

In linear tomography a) Blurring is the distortion of definition of objects out-side the focal plane. b) The fulcrum is the pivot point about which the lever arm rotates. It determines the plane that will be in focus. c) The focal plane is the plane of maximal focus, and represents the axis (fulcrum) about which the X-ray tube and film rotate. d) The focal plane level is the height of the focal plane above the tabletop. e) The tomographic angle or arc is the amplitude of tube travel expressed in degrees. f) The exposure angle is the angle through which the X-ray beam (or central ray) moves during the exposure.

As the tube and film move from the first position to the second, all points in the focal plane project to the same position on X-ray film. Thus, points x, y and z project to points x', y' and z' in the first position and x", y" and z" in the second position (Figs 25.3A and B). Points above or below the focal plane do not project to the same film positions and are blurred. By changing the relative motion of the film and tube, the focal plane can be adjusted upward or downward.

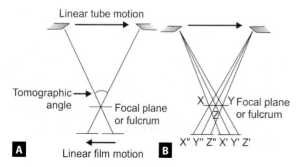

Figs 25.3A and B X-ray linear tomography

Working

The tube and film/detector are linked by an extensible rod, hinged about a pivot. During exposure, the film/detector moves in a straight line, e.g. left-to-right along rails, whilst the tube moves the other way. While moving, the tube is rotated so that the central ray always points toward the pivot point. Structures that are in the same plane as pivot point (focal plane) will not move when projected onto the film, producing a sharp image. The projections of structures outside the focal plane will move around on the film, and hence are blurred in the final image. The further the object is from the focal plane, the greater is the blurring. Cut-height (the focal plane position) is adjusted by lowering or raising the pivot.

SOFT TISSUE RADIOGRAPHY

Soft tissue radiography is a modified conventional radiography technique used for imaging of soft tissues of the body without use of contrast media. Soft tissue radiography is commonly done by using low kVp technique, minimum filtration of beam and with the use of special Molybdenum target in mammography. Soft tissues have low tissue densities and low X-ray absorptive ability and therefore tissues including tendons, ligaments, adipose tissue and cartilage, are not visible, for any practical purposes, with conventional radiography.

Soft tissue radiography is used for
- Mammography
- Low density foreign bodies
- Air in soft tissues
- Soft tissue changes adjacent to bone pathology
- Calcification in soft tissues
- The adenoids
- Fatty lesions
- Cysticercosis
- larynx

Following points to be considered while performing soft tissue radiography,
- *Optimum radiographic contrast* is achieved using appropriate exposure technique and by reducing scatter radiation. Appropriate exposure technique is achieved by means of normal kVp and low kVp techniques and minimum filtration of beam. Normal kVp technique achieves optimum contrast using natural contrast of air shadow and fat delineating abnormalities in soft tissues. Normal kVp technique also achieves contrast by using wedge filter and nonscreen and a film screen combination. Low kVp technique generates low energy beam and hence improves the contrast of soft tissues. Maximum contrast will be achieved if

the lowest possible kVp is used which will allow a reasonable proportion of the radiation to penetrate the body part. All added filtration must be removed in order to use the lowest energy radiation for contrast enhancement.

Optimum contrast in mammography is achieved by use of molybdenum (Mo) target. At about 80kV Mo target emit characteristic radiation in the range of 17.4 and 19.5 kV which is optimum for soft tissue radiography. In addition Mo filters are used in mammography to remove much of radiation with energy above and below the desired range, thereby producing a nearly monoenergetic beam.

Scatter radiation decreases the image contrast. In the low energy range (20 to 30 keV), in which the photoelectric effect predominates, extremely little scatter radiation is produced. As the radiation energy increases, the percentage of Compton reactions increases, and so does the production of scatter radiation.

- *Image sharpness:* Geometric or focal spot blur is reduced by use of small focal spot size, long focus film distance (FFD), and short object film distance (OFD). Motion blur is reduced by careful immobilization of the part to be radiographed, exposure for short time, and use of intensifying screens.
- *Reducing artifacts:* Reduction of artifacts in radiographed image produced secondary to storage of films, handling of unexposed films, artifacts produced during exposure as well as during development of film improves the image quality and hence soft tissue visualization.

A novel X-ray technology, called diffraction enhanced imaging (DEI) has been developed for soft tissue radiography. DEI is capable of rendering images with absorption, refraction and scatter rejection qualities and allows detection of specific soft tissues based on small differences in tissue densities. DEI allows high contrast imaging of soft tissues, including ligaments, tendons and adipose tissue, of the human foot and ankle. DEI uses a synchrotron X-ray source. The strength of the technology is that it utilizes a series of perfect silicon crystals to provide images with enhanced contrast depending on the extent of X-ray ultra small angle scattering and refraction by the object.

DENTAL FILM

The film used in dental radiography is composed of fexible, thin polyster plastic base. The base is coated on each side by emulsion and is attached firmly by an adhesive. The emulsion is made of homogenous crystals of silver halide mixed in gelatin. The size of

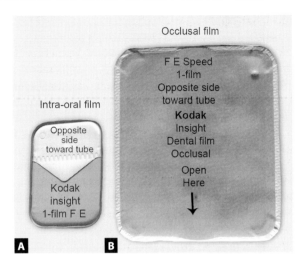

Figs 25.4A and B Dental film and occlusal film
(*For color version, see Plate 8*)

crystal in emulsion regulate the speed of film. Larger the crystal faster is the film. Film speeds available for dental radiography are D-speed, E-speed and F-speed, with D-speed being the slowest and F-speed the fastest. The use of faster film speed can result in up to a 50% decrease in exposure to the patient without compromising diagnostic quality.

There are two types of films intraoral (direct action) film and extra oral (screen) film. Intraoral films are small, double-emulsion films without screens wrapped in a black paper with a lead foil backing to reduce patient dose, enclosed in a moisture-resistant plastic envelope (Fig. 25.4A). The occlusal film (Fig. 25.4B), which is about three to four times the size of other intraoral films, is inserted into the mouth so as to entirely separate the maxillary and mandibular teeth, and the film is exposed either from under the chin or angled down from the top of the nose. Extra oral films are large, single-emulsion, screen films.

MOBILE RADIOGRAPHY

It is also called "portable" or "bed-side" imaging. It is the general term covering all X-ray examinations made by "mobile" X-ray units, in combination with screen-film detectors, digital detectors or C-arms. In most institutions mobile radiography is still performed with conventional screen-film systems. However, digital techniques are taking over rapidly.

Three classes of digital mobile radiography devices can be distinguished:

1. Digital off-line detectors for digital mobile radiography are exclusively the field of computed radiography (CR), which is based upon "stimulable phosphor" plates, mounted in a modified conventional cassette. This cassette can be placed

behind the patient, with or without grid and uses the same exposure techniques and equipment as the conventional screen-film systems.

2. *C-arms:* Offer the advantage of fluoroscopy but lack field of view and image quality. Their application is limited to surgery wards and emergency rooms. Many "digital" C-arms are video-based systems.

3. Digital on-line systems with solid state detectors (such as amorphous selenium or silicon) exist but are not yet in use for digital mobile radiography. These detectors are still too bulky and vulnerable to mechanical damage and need a cable connection to the network or monitor as well as to the X-ray unit for steering.

Computed radiography (CR) uses a robust inexpensive cassette off-line from the reading unit, which can be used for other X-ray work. The stimulable memory phosphors do not require films, but keep the image stored until they are digitized in a reader and can be re-used up to 10,000 times. Over- and underexposure is virtually excluded and produces a stable and excellent image quality independent of exposure technique, dose and patient, allowing an easy day-by-day comparison of chest images. Digital mobile radiography adopts all current exposure techniques ranging from low kVp without grid to high kVp with grid. The image processing behind CR is a necessary component in digital mobile radiography, because it enables a better visualization of the typical problems in intensive care chest radiology.

FILM BADGE

The film badge dosimeter, or film badge, is a dosimeter used for monitoring cumulative exposure to ionizing radiation. The badge consists of two parts: photographic film or dental X-ray film and a holder. The film is removed and developed to measure exposure. The film badge is used to measure and record radiation exposure due to gamma rays, X-rays and beta particles. The film is packaged in a light proof, vapour proof envelope preventing light, moisture or chemical vapours from affecting the film. A special film is used which is coated with two different emulsions. One side is coated with a large grain, fast emulsion that is sensitive to low levels of exposure. The other side of the film is coated with a fine grain, slow emulsion that is less sensitive to exposure. The combination of a low-sensitivity and high-sensitivity emulsion extends the dynamic range to several orders of magnitude. The film is backed by a sheet of lead foil to absorb radiation from behind the badge. The film is contained inside a film holder or badge. The badge incorporates a series of filters to determine the quality of the radiation. To monitor gamma rays or X-rays, the filters are metal,

usually tin or lead. To monitor beta particle emission, the filters use various densities of plastic. The badge holder also contains an open window to determine radiation exposure due to beta particles. Beta particles are effectively shielded by a thin amount of material. The major advantages of a film badge as a personnel monitoring device are that it provides a permanent record, it is able to distinguish between different energies of photons and it can measure doses due to different types of radiation. It is quite accurate for exposures greater than 100 millirem. The major disadvantages are that it must be developed and read by a processor (which is time consuming), prolonged heat exposure can affect the film and exposures of less than 20 millirem of gamma radiation cannot be accurately measured. Film badges need to be worn correctly so that the dose they receive accurately represents the dose the wearer receives. Whole body badges are worn on the body between the neck and the waist, often on the belt or a shirt pocket. Pregnant women should wear a second badge over abdomen beneath the leaded apron. The clip-on badge is worn most often when performing X-ray or gamma radiography. Usually the badges are returned after one month and dosimetric comparison is made with standard films exposed to known amounts of radiation.

THERMOLUMINESCENCE DOSIMETER BADGE

A thermo luminescence dosimeter (TLD) measures ionizing radiation exposure by measuring the amount of visible light emitted from crystal in the detector when the crystal is heated (Fig. 25.5). The amount of light emitted is dependent upon the radiation

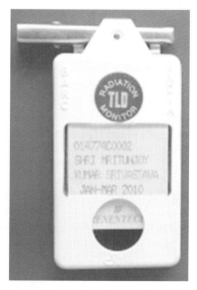

Fig. 25.5 Thermoluminescent dosimeters

exposure. Materials exhibiting thermo luminescence in response to ionizing radiation include calcium fluoride, calcium sulfate, calcium borate, lithium fluoride, lithium borate, potassium bromide, and feldspar. When a TLD is exposed to ionizing radiation at ambient temperatures, the radiation interacts with the phosphor crystal and deposits all or part of the incident energy in that material. Some of the atoms in the material that absorb that energy become ionized, producing free electrons and areas lacking one or more electrons, called holes. Imperfections in the crystal lattice structure act as sites where free electrons can become trapped and locked into place.

Heating the crystal causes the crystal lattice to vibrate, releasing the trapped electrons in the process. Released electrons return to the original ground state, releasing the captured energy from ionization as light, hence the name thermo luminescent. Released light is counted using photomultiplier tubes and the number of photons counted is proportional to the quantity of radiation striking the phosphor.

Thermoluminescent dosimeters (TLD) are often used instead of the film badge (Fig. 25.5). Like a film badge, it is worn for a period of time (usually 3 months or less) and then must be processed to determine the dose received, if any. Thermoluminescent dosimeters can measure doses as low as 1 millirem. The advantages of a TLD over other personnel monitors are its linearity of response to dose, its relative energy independence, and its sensitivity to low doses. It is also reusable, which is an advantage over film badges. However, no permanent record or re-readability is provided and an immediate, on the job readout is not possible.

MASS MINIATURE RADIOGRAPHY

Mass miniature radiography (MMR) is a technique of rapid screening by X-rays to pick up infectious disease such as pulmonary tuberculosis (TB). Using a cassette with a roll of film 70 mm wide, radiographers could take many films using a low dose of radiation. These were read centrally by radiologists and if there was any doubt, patients were recalled for a full chest film.

The smaller size of the equipment meant that it could be mounted in a van and taken to schools and workplaces.

In many countries, miniature mass radiographs (MMR) was quickly adopted and extensively utilized in the 1950s. However, as a mass screening program for low-risk populations, the procedure was largely discontinued in the 1970s, following recommendation of the World Health Organization, due to three main reasons:

The dramatic decrease of the general incidence of tuberculosis in developed countries.
1. Decreased benefits/cost ratio.
2. Risk of exposure to ionizing radiation doses, particularly among children, in the presence of extremely low yield rates of detection.
3. MMR is still an easy and useful way to prevent transmission of the disease in certain situations, such as in prisons and for immigration applicants and foreign workers coming from countries with a higher risk for tuberculosis.

MMR is most useful at detecting tuberculosis infection in the asymptomatic phase and it should be combined with tuberculin skin tests and clinical questioning in order to be more effective. The sharp increase in tuberculosis in all countries with large exposure to HIV is probably mandating a return of MMR as a screening tool focusing on high-risk populations, such as homosexuals and intravenous drug users.

RADIATION UNITS

Radiation is energy in transit in the form of high speed particles and electromagnetic waves. Radiation can be ionizing or nonionizing. X-rays are electromagnetic waves or photons not emitted from the nucleus, but normally emitted by energy changes in electrons. These energy changes are either in electron orbital shells that surround an atom or in the process of slowing down such as in an X-ray machine.

Roentgen is a unit used to measure a quantity called exposure. One roentgen is equal to depositing in dry air enough energy to cause 2.58×10^{-4} coulombs per kg. It is a measure of the ionizations of the molecules in a mass of air.

Radiation absorbed dose (RAD) is a unit used to measure a quantity called absorbed dose. This relates to the amount of energy actually absorbed in some material, and is used for any type of radiation and any material. One rad is defined as the absorption of 100 ergs per gram of material.

Roentgen equivalent man (REM) is a unit used to derive a quantity called equivalent dose. This relates the absorbed dose in human tissue to the effective biological damage of the radiation. Equivalent dose is often expressed in terms of thousandths of a rem, or mrem. To determine equivalent dose (rem), you multiply absorbed dose (rad) by a quality factor (Q) that is unique to the type of incident radiation.

Curie (Ci) is a unit used to measure a radioactivity. One curie is that quantity of a radioactive material that will have 37,000,000,000 transformations in one second. The relationship between Becquerel and curies is: 3.7×10^{10} Bq in one curie.

Gray (Gy) is a unit used to measure a quantity called absorbed dose. This relates to the amount of energy actually absorbed in some material, and is used for any type of radiation and any material. One gray is equal to one joule of energy deposited in one kg of a material. Absorbed dose is often expressed in terms of hundredths of a gray, or centi-grays. One gray is equivalent to 100 rads.

Sievert (Sv) is a unit used to derive a quantity called equivalent dose. This relates the absorbed dose in human tissue to the effective biological damage of the radiation. Equivalent dose is often expressed in terms of millionths of a sievert, or micro-sievert. To determine equivalent dose (Sv), you multiply absorbed dose (Gy) by a quality factor (Q) that is unique to the type of incident radiation. One sievert is equivalent to 100 rem. 1 Sv = 1,000,000 μSv, mSv = 10,000 μSv.

Becquerel (Bq) is a unit used to measure a radioactivity. One Becquerel is that quantity of a radioactive material that will have 1 transformation in one second. Often radioactivity is expressed in larger units like: thousands (k Bq), one millions (m Bq) or even billions (g Bq) of a Becquerel. As a result of having one Becquerel being equal to one transformation per second, there are 3.7×10^{10} Bq in one curie.

GAMMA RAYS

Gamma-rays (γ) are electromagnetic radiations of high frequency. They are very high energy ionizing radiation and are thus biologically hazardous. Gamma photons have about 10,000 times as much energy as the photons in the visible range of the electromagnetic spectrum. They have no mass and no electrical charge, they are pure electromagnetic energy. Because of their high energy, they travel at the speed of light and can cover hundreds to thousands of meters in air before spending their energy. They can pass through many kinds of materials, including human tissue. Very dense materials, such as lead, are commonly used as shielding to slow or stop gamma photons. They are classically produced by the decay from high energy states of atomic nuclei (gamma decay), but also in many other ways. Natural sources of gamma rays on Earth include gamma decay from naturally-occurring radioisotopes such as potassium-40, and also as a secondary radiation from various atmospheric interactions with cosmic ray particles. Some rare terrestrial natural sources produce gamma rays that are not of a nuclear origin are lightning strikes and terrestrial gamma-ray flashes, which produce high energy emissions from natural high-energy voltages. Gamma rays are produced by a number of astronomical processes in which very high-energy electrons are produced.

Medical applications of gamma rays include the valuable imaging technique of positron emission tomography (PET) and effective radiation therapies to treat cancerous tumors.

In a PET scan, a short-lived positron-emitting radioactive pharmaceutical is chosen because of its participation in a particular physiological process (e.g. brain function), is injected into the body. Emitted positrons quickly combine with nearby electrons and, through pair annihilation, give rise to two 511-keV gamma rays traveling in opposite directions. After detection of the gamma rays, a computer-generated reconstruction of the locations of the gamma-ray emissions produces an image that highlights the location of the biological process being examined.

As a deeply penetrating ionizing radiation, gamma rays cause significant biochemical changes in living cells. Radiation therapies make use of this property to selectively destroy cancerous cells in small localized tumors. Radioactive isotopes are injected or implanted near the tumor; gamma rays that are continuously emitted by the radioactive nuclei bombard the affected area and arrest the development of the malignant cells.

Gamma rays cause cell damage and can cause a variety of cancers. They cause mutations in growing tissues, so unborn babies are especially vulnerable.

XERORADIOGRAPHY

Xeroradiography is the science of recording radiographic images electronically. Xeroradiography is the production of a visible image from an X-ray exposure utilizing the charged surface of a photoconductor (amorphous selenium) as the X-ray detecting medium.

Xeroradiography is a complex electro-static process based on a special material called a photoconductor. A photoconductor will not conduct an electric current when shielded from radiation, but becomes conductive when exposed to radiation such as visible light or X-rays. The photoconductor used in xeroradiography is amorphous selenium. The selenium layer is semiconductive. The selenium is deposited as a thin layer onto a sheet of aluminum to form the xeroradiographic plate, which is analogous to film used in conventional radiography. A very thin aluminum oxide layer is placed as an electric insulator between the selenium and the conducting aluminum plate. The plate is enclosed in a light-tight cassette.

The xeroradiographic imaging process consists of several steps:
- A uniform charge is deposited onto the surface of the selenium. This sensitizes the plate before exposure to X-rays.
- The charged plate is placed in a light-tight cassette and exposed to X-rays. X-rays reaching the plate

cause the photo-conductor layer to lose its charge in an amount corresponding to the intensity of the X-ray beam. The uniform charge is thus partly dissipated and the remaining charge pattern forms the latent electrostatic image.

- The latent electrostatic image is developed (made visible) by exposing the surface of the plate to fine-charged particles (called "toner") that are attracted to the plate surface in proportion to the intensity of the remaining charge.
- The toner image is transferred to a receiver sheet by an electrostatic process.
- The toner image is fixed to the sheet to make a permanent record.
- The plate is cleaned of all remaining toner and prepared for reuse. The plate is not charged during storage.

The advantages of xeroradiography include the following:

- Greater diagnostic accuracy is possible;
- Interpretation is easier and more rapidly achieved;
- The radiographic work is simplified and there is the assurance of good quality images;
- Exposure times are shorter and there is consequently less patient movement
- A relatively low radiation dose.

Xeroradiography has been used most extensively for bones, soft tissue and mammography applications.

A higher sensitivity Xerox system, the 175 System reduces exposure factors for to about half those previously required. It is more sensitive photoreceptor which is achieved by thicker layer and greater conversion efficiency and higher sensitivity development by introducing liquid toner with smaller particles.

Unfortunately, inspite of low dose efficiency for xeroradiography systems it has not achieved high utilization.

P VALUE

In statistical significance testing, the p-value or calculated probability is the estimated probability of rejecting the null hypothesis (H0) of a study question when that hypothesis is true. The null hypothesis is usually an hypothesis of "no difference". One often "rejects the null hypothesis" when the p-value is less than the significance level α, which is often 0.05 or 0.01. When the null hypothesis is rejected, the result is said to be statistically significant. Most authors refer to statistically significant as $P < 0.05$ and statistically highly significant as $P < 0.001$. The p-value remains the most widely utilized tool to draw inference from medical studies.

Sensitivity

The sensitivity of a clinical test refers to the ability of the test to correctly identify those patients with the disease.

$$\text{Sensitivity} = \frac{\text{True positives}}{\text{True positives} + \text{False negatives}}$$

If a test has high sensitivity then a negative result would suggest the absence of disease.

Specificity

The specificity of a clinical test refers to the ability of the test to correctly identify those patients without the disease.

$$\text{Specificity} = \frac{\text{True negatives}}{\text{True negatives} + \text{False positives}}$$

If a test has high specificity, a positive result from the test means a high probability of the presence of disease.

Positive Predictive Value

'How likely is it that the patient has the disease given that the test result is positive?'

$$\text{Positive predictive value} = \frac{\text{True positives}}{\text{True positives} + \text{False positives}}$$

Negative Predictive Value

'How likely is it that the patient does not have the disease given that the test result is negative?'

$$\text{Negative predictive value} = \frac{\text{True negatives}}{\text{True negatives} + \text{False negatives}}$$

Angiographic Catheters

A catheter is a hollow, tubular, flexible tube that can be inserted into a body cavity, duct or vessel. Catheters allow drainage or injection of fluids, distend a passageway or provide access by surgical instruments. The process of inserting a catheter is catheterization.

Angiographic catheters are one through which a contrast medium is injected for visualization of the vascular system of an organ. They come in multiple preformed shapes, the cobra, sidewinder, headhunter (Fig. 25.6) for selective angiography, and pigtail configuration for nonselective flush angiograms being the most common.

Microcatheters are low profile catheters 1F to 3F which can be advanced through angiographic catheters 4F to 6F for super-selective catheterization and embolization.

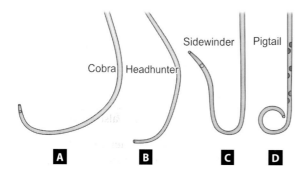

Figs 25.6A to D Angiographic catheters in multiple preformed shapes (A) The cobra; (B) Headhunter; (C) Sidewinder; (D) Pigtail for selective angiography

Balloon catheters contain one or multiple lumina through which one or more attached balloons can be inflated. An additional lumen usually serves for introduction of guidewires for flushing and contrast injection. Flow directed balloon catheters are taken to the periphery by the blood stream. Occlusion balloon catheters are used to occlude a vessel for diagnostic or therapeutic purposes.

Dilatation catheters have balloons made usually from noncompliant material such as polyethylene, etc. to guarantee high resistance and high burst pressures.

Drainage catheters have one or more (usually 2 to 3) lumina where a thinner lumen and are used for flushing and a larger for drainage.

CLOUD COMPUTING

The National Institute of Standards and Technology (NIST) has presented the clearest and most comprehensive definition of cloud computing. Cloud computing is a model for enabling convenient, on-demand network access to a shared pool of configurable computing resources which includes networks, servers, storage, applications, and services, that can be rapidly provisioned and released with minimal management effort or service provider interaction. This cloud model promotes availability and is composed of essential characteristics, deployment models, and various service models. The Institute categorizes cloud computing into 5 key categories: on-demand self-service, ubiquitous network access, location-independent resource pooling, rapid elasticity, and measured service. Cloud technologies can also be deployed as private, community, public, or hybrid clouds. Private clouds are operated for a specific organization, and are more popular in healthcare, whereas community clouds are shared by a number of organizations.

Cloud technologies in imaging can reduce capital expenditures on hardware in particular, but also in software and services, especially when deployed on a wider scale.

Radiology is increasingly dealing with large imaging data sets, complex algorithms, pre- and postprocessing requirements and an increasingly distributed environment. Distributed data grids perform much more efficiently compared to hard drives, primarily because memory is shared between data centers. Hence, performance is better. Deployments can also be more effectively and consistently managed across the healthcare enterprise, freeing users from the finer details of IT system configuration and maintenance, allowing them to focus instead on care delivery.

In this era of distributed digital imaging, there are specific needs for radiologists to have the ability not just to access images at the point of care, but also to be able to work efficiently and effectively from multiple locations, with full access to the complete imaging data sets, relevant priors, relevant clinical information, as well as to the right set of diagnostic tools, from any location. Cloud-based deployments provide a more robust and sophisticated security strategy.

With digital revolution in radiology, it is resulting in more CDs and DVDs of patient studies than ever before. The future imaging department will have to deal a lot more intelligently with data and information explosion. With increase in the digital-imaging in healthcare, the data is growing from terabytes to petabytes. (1 megabyte - 10^6 byte, 1 gigabyte – 10^9 byte, 1 terabyte – 10^{12} byte, 1 petabyte – 10^{15} byte). Cloud computing offers ways for these challenges, with more actionable data and knowledge of information systems, across healthcare enterprise.

ULTRASOUND WIRELESS TRANSDUCERS

Normally a transducer is connected to the ultrasound system via a cable. This setup sharply restricts the operator's freedom of movement. In addition the controls on the ultrasound unit are not sterile and in some cases need to be operated by a second technician.

It eliminates the need of cables and provides easier and more flexible scanning because there is no cable tethering the system and transducers together. Freedom from cable weight or torque allows for greater ease in obtaining accurate transducer and needle positioning during invasive procedures.

Wireless transducers provides real time wireless imaging and prevents interface with other electronic equipments. Multiple antennas on the transducer and system dedicated to high speed data transmission. Build in transducer controls allow easy access to real time operating functions. The user can operate upto nine feet away from the main system which is longer than a cabled device.

To reduce the amount of data transferred between the transducer and the system without degrading the image quality, the system uses synthetic aperture technology. With this technology each individual pixel in the image is digitally focused once it's been transmitted to the console. As opposed to the traditional acoustic transmit focusing method, which requires users to manually focus on a region of interest, the synthetic focusing provides automatic uniform focusing throughout the entire field of view resulting in a superior image quality.

Elimination of cables is particularly helpful in operations or during invasive procedures in which the needle visualization needs to be monitored using ultrasound technology.

The wireless transducers are lightweight, ergonomic and rechargeable, uses a lithium ion battery which lasts for 90 minutes of total scanning time. Wireless alert system helps keep track on transducer locations.

These transducers are easy to sterile with reduced risk of contaminating the sterile field during guided procedure.

Index

Page numbers followed by *f* refer to figure and *t* refer to table